ORGAN
TRANSPLANTATION

ORGAN
TRANSPLANTATION

David Petechuk

Health and Medical Issues Today

GREENWOOD PRESS
Westport, Connecticut • London

Library of Congress Cataloging-in-Publication Data

Petechuk, David.
    Organ transplantation / David Petechuk.
       p. cm. — (Health and medical issues today, ISSN 1558–7592)
    Includes bibliographical references and index.
    ISBN 0–313–33542–7 (alk. paper)
    1. Transplantation of organs, tissues, etc.   I. Title.
  RD120.7.P46   2006
  617.9'5—dc22   2006021342

British Library Cataloguing in Publication Data is available.

Library of Congress Catalog Card Number: 2006021342
ISBN: 0–313–33542–7
ISSN: 1558–7592

First published in 2006

Greenwood Press, 88 Post Road West, Westport, CT 06881
An imprint of Greenwood Publishing Group, Inc.
www.greenwood.com

Printed in the United States of America

The paper used in this book complics with the
Permanent Paper Standard issued by the National
Information Standards Organization (Z39.48–1984).

10 9 8 7 6 5 4 3 2 1

Every reasonable effort has been made to trace the owners of copyright materials in this
book, but in some instances this has proven impossible. The author and publisher will be
glad to receive information leading to more complete acknowledgments in subsequent
printings of the book and in the meantime extend their apologies for any omissions.

CONTENTS

Section Three   References and Resources

SERIES FOREWORD

Every day, the public is bombarded with information on developments in medicine and health care. Whether it is on the latest techniques in treatments or research, or on concerns over public health threats, this information directly impacts the lives of people more than almost any other issue. Although there are many sources for understanding these topics—from Web sites and blogs to newspapers and magazines—students and ordinary citizens often need one resource that makes sense of the complex health and medical issues affecting their daily lives.

The *Health and Medical Issues Today* series provides just such a one-stop resource for obtaining a solid overview of the most controversial areas of health care today. Each volume addresses one topic and provides a balanced summary of what is known. These volumes provide an excellent first step for students and lay people interested in understanding how health care works in our society today.

Each volume is broken into several sections to provide readers and researchers with easy access to the information they need:

- Section I provides overview chapters on background information—including chapters on such areas as the historical, scientific, medical, social, and legal issues involved—that a citizen needs to intelligently understand the topic.
- Section II provides capsule examinations of the most heated contemporary issues and debates, and analyzes in a balanced manner the viewpoints held by various advocates in the debates.

- Section III provides a selection of reference material, including annotated primary source documents, a timeline of important events, and an annotated bibliography of useful print and electronic resources that serve as the best next step in learning about the topic at hand.

The *Health and Medical Issues Today* series strives to provide readers with all the information needed to begin making sense of some of the most important debates going on in the world today. The series will include volumes on such topics as stem-cell research, obesity, gene therapy, alternative medicine, organ transplantation, mental health, and more.

PREFACE

The debates and controversies discussed in *Organ Transplantation* focus on longtime, fundamental issues in the field, such as the shortage of organ donors and the responsibility to make sure that a scarce lifesaving resource is allocated appropriately. New advances in the expanding field of transplantation also come under inspection. Embryonic stem cell transplantation, for example, may be many years away from becoming a viable therapy. Nevertheless, current ethical concerns are important because they could ultimately decide whether society pursues this controversial therapy, which encompasses debates involving personal religious beliefs and questions about when "life" begins. Face transplantation, on the other hand, is much closer to becoming a reality, yet questions have been raised over the procedure's psychological impacts and the potentially serious health risks associated with the potent immunological drugs patients will likely have to take for the rest of their lives.

Another area of transplantation engenders questions concerning the prospect of potentially harming a healthy person to help another. Is it appropriate for society and the medical establishment to foster live organ donation, even if the person appears to want to donate? Sanctioning live organ donation might place undue societal pressures on people to donate, especially family members. Furthermore, live donation might benefit the wealthy at the expense of the poor and others, especially if some type of payment is made to donors. Xenotransplantation (the transplanting of organs and tissues across species) is a developing area of transplantation that was once relegated to the realms of science fiction and fantasy. Recent advances, however, have led to ethical and practical ponderings as old as animal rights issues and as new as the possibility of spreading a deadly virus into the human population.

In today's world of mass media and instant communications, the general public is better informed about almost every aspect of society. Of course, even today's media is surrounded in controversy, often accused of having a "liberal" bias or "conservative" bent depending on the source of information. Even though much of the information in this book has been culled from a variety of sources, from medical and ethics journals to newspaper articles and the Internet, this volume seeks to bring together in one readily available resource information on some of the most prominent controversies surrounding several areas of transplantation. The ultimate goal is to provide a balanced overview of both sides of the debates and, secondarily, to give readers a basic foundation in the history of the field and background on current issues. Although it is important to understand the "science" of transplantation, the science presented in *Organ Transplantation* is primarily limited to advances and procedures that impact or influence a debate.

INTRODUCTION

British philosopher and social critic Bertrand Russell once noted, "Change is scientific, progress is ethical; change is indubitable, whereas progress is a matter of controversy." In the case of transplantation, few would dispute that the field has had many proven benefits in caring for the terminally ill or that future progress can change even more lives for the better. Organ transplantation offers the hope of life for people suffering from a wide range of diseases that lead to end-stage organ failure and death. Many believe that the development of new transplantation specialties, such as stem cell transplantation, will also give new hope one day for millions suffering from cancer, spinal cord injuries, neurological disorders such as Parkinson's disease, and a host of other debilitating and often deadly maladies. Recent efforts to pursue face transplantation are also viewed by some as having the near miraculous potential to ease the horrendous, long-term psychological burdens experienced by people with severe disfigurements.

Despite all these positives, controversy has surrounded transplantation almost every step of the way in its development. Although organ transplantation today is considered a viable lifesaving therapy, the field struggled for decades to achieve legitimacy. In the early days, often referred to as "the black years," transplant recipients routinely died because of the high failure rates of the organs transplanted. By 1963, for example, approximately two-thirds of all transplant recipients, not counting transplants between identical twins, died from organ rejection. Approximately two decades passed before new immunosuppressive drugs moved transplantation beyond the realm of "experimental." Until that time, transplant pioneers were routinely ridiculed by some of their medical colleagues, and many believed that the research time and effort put into advancing the field would be better applied to other "more promising" aspects of medicine and patient care.

Although organ transplantation has become a viable and widely accepted therapy, controversy still surrounds the field. Ironically, most of the controversies and ethical dilemmas associated with organ transplantation have resulted from the field's phenomenal success. Today, more than 90,000 people in the United States alone are waiting for a transplant. Unfortunately, as the United Network for Organ Sharing (UNOS) transplant waiting list grows each year, more and more people die because an organ is not available for transplantation. In 2005, nearly 6,000 people died while waiting for a donor organ that never materialized. As a result, controversy surrounds how such precious lifesaving resources are and should be allocated.

Some have proposed developing an economically based market system for the sale of organs to increase donation rates whereas others see any move away from the altruistic notion of organ donation as a "gift of life" as being fraught with ethical dilemmas. The use of living donors is another issue, with some perceiving the use of living donors as being contrary to the basic dictum for physicians to "do no harm." Is it right, some ask, for the medical establishment to risk the health and lives of healthy people to help others? Another effort to increase the supply of organs, namely the transplantation of organs from animals to humans (xenotransplantation), involves questions of our identity as humans and fears over the potential to introduce new and deadly viral diseases into the population.

Stem cell transplantation, specifically embryonic stem cell transplantation, has led to a national debate following restrictions placed by President George W. Bush on federal funding for such research. One side of the debate sees a huge upside to research with these cells, which can morph into almost any type of cell. Advocates of embryonic stem cell research believe the field holds the key for the treatment and potential cure of a variety of insidious, debilitating, and potentially fatal diseases that have so far resisted the best efforts of science to find a cure. A "pro-life" contingent, however, argues that these cells are "potential" human lives and that using them is the equivalent of taking a life. Basing their beliefs on both religious and ethical grounds, they argue that taking one life to save another is always wrong.

Like stem cell transplantation, facial transplantation is still in the early stages of development, with the determination of its ultimate success or failure perhaps still many years away. Nevertheless, partial face transplants by a group of French surgeons in 2005 and by Chinese surgeons in 2006 have raised ethical concerns as the prospect of a full face transplant approaches. Some fear that the transplants would ultimately be little more than a mask at best and eventually could be rejected, leaving the recipients—who have already suffered severe emotional turmoil—even worse off than before. Many also debate whether the long-term health risks associated with a lifetime of immunosuppression therapy are warranted, considering that, unlike organ transplantation, face transplants are not necessary to save a person's life.

The modern era of health care has brought many "miraculous" treatments or cures for a host of diseases and medical problems that have plagued humankind throughout its history. Many of the medical tools and treatments routinely used today were once seen as controversial, such as the development of anesthesia in the mid-1800s. Some people at the time argued against its use in obstetrics because of questions concerning the mother's and the fetus's safety, and others based their objections on a theology that said altering the birthing process in any way is against God and nature. Today, of course, anesthesia is used routinely for birthing and for almost all invasive surgical procedures. Yet this does not mean that the controversies raised in the past were invalid. As rational human beings it is our duty to question before entering the unknown, especially when a medical or technical advance has the potential to profoundly impact human life in either a positive or a negative way—or perhaps both.

As Bertrand Russell pointed out, progress and change, whether in medicine and science or in society in general, are almost always controversial. The unknown inevitably raises questions, and as a society we seek answers. Sometimes ethical questions and dilemmas remain intractable; otherwise, they would not remain issues for long. Oftentimes, personal beliefs, whether in religion, in a social norm, or in some other belief system, are the deciding factors that lead an individual to come down on one side of the argument or the other. In other instances, science may come up with a solution. For example, researchers could develop a therapy using nonembryonic stem cells, which would effectively end the debate from the transplantation standpoint. This book contains no solutions, and in the end it may be as twentieth-century writer and social critic James Thurber noted: "It is better to know some of the questions than all of the answers."

SECTION ONE

Overview

CHAPTER 1

A Brief History of Transplantation

In an article commemorating the fiftieth anniversary of the first successful organ transplant in the United States, transplantation pioneer Thomas E. Starzl remarked, "The growth of transplantation from ground zero to its present state seems like a fairy tale, a fantasy that became reality because of the courage of our patients. The truth is that none of us in the 1950's remotely envisioned the height to which transplantation would rise and the way it has changed the face of medicine" (Altman, *New York Times*, 2004).

Starzl and his transplantation colleagues had good reason to keep their vision for transplantation tempered in the early days. The specter of organ rejection and patient death loomed over the field from the very beginning, and those toiling to develop it had to steel themselves against doubters and naysayers, a group including many of their colleagues in medicine and surgery. Ethical issues and questions were raised from the start. Anti-vivisectionists in the early twentieth century opposed surgical experimentations with animals. Prohibitions in some religions and societies treated transplantation as a defilement of the sacred human body. Failure and disappointments were common, leading many in the medical profession to question whether transplants could ever work. When transplantation became a reality in the latter half of the twentieth century, transplant specialists were then accused of "playing God" by deciding who would receive an organ and, thus, who would live or die.

Although ethical debates associated with transplantation continue, transplantation is recognized worldwide as an established therapy that saves lives. Still, those in the transplant field realize that there is still more

The Father of Transplantation

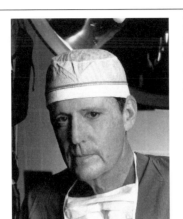

(Photo courtesy of Dr. Starzl.)

Many surgeons and medical researchers have made important contributions to the advancement of transplantation. Few, however, have had such a wide-ranging impact on the field as Thomas E. Starzl. His clinical, scientific, and ethical contributions to the field of transplantation have rightly earned him the designation among many as the "Father of Transplantation."

Throughout his career, Starzl made some of the most important landmark advancements in transplantation. He performed the first human liver transplant in 1963 and the first successful liver transplant in 1967. He introduced many of the immunosuppression regimens that allowed transplantation to become successful, including the clinical use of anti-lymphocyte globulin and cyclosporine in 1980, which is considered the major step that advanced transplantation from an experimental procedure to an accepted form of treatment. Although he retired from performing transplants in 1991, Starzl has continued to head important research in such areas as cross-species transplantation and transplant tolerance. He introduced the concept of microchimerism, a state in which the coexistence of donor and recipient cells may lead to a better understanding of transplant organ acceptance and a crucial step in the development of whole organ tolerance without the need for immunosuppressive drugs, which have many serious side effects.

Starzl's efforts have also focused on the ethical and societal implications of transplantation. He led the efforts that resulted in a 1984 National Institutes of Health consensus conference that approved liver transplantation as a therapeutic modality for the treatment of end-stage liver disease. He and his colleagues at the University of Pittsburgh, where he was recruited in 1981, also played a lead role in the process to change the United Network for Organ Sharing (UNOS) organ allocation policies and make the transplant allocation system fairer for recipients.

> The authors of *1,000 Years, 1000 People* named Starzl as one of the "1,000 men and women who, over the course of the past 1,000 years, did the most to shape the world" (Gottlieb et al., 1998). Even more important, however, is the list compiled by the Institute for Scientific Information (ISI) and published in the May/June 1999 issue of *ScienceWatch*. The ISI noted that Starzl had the most impact on clinical medicine between the years of 1981 and 1998, as evidenced by his number-one ranking in the number of times a researcher's publications were cited by other researchers. Starzl was the most cited researcher in journals of clinical medicine, with 26,456 citations, about 4,000 more times than the second-ranked researcher. According to ISI, Starzl once averaged one paper every 7.3 days, making him one of the most prolific published scientists in the world.

to do to improve the field. In his memoir *The Puzzle People*, Starzl commented on the successes he and others had achieved and noted, "To have the fog lift, exposing this clarifying vision, was like being allowed a glimpse of eternity. The moment of tranquility that followed was a fair trade for the thirty-five years of work preceding it. And then it was gone, banished by the next set of questions" (Starzl, 1992).

AN ANCIENT IDEA?

The idea of people sharing body parts among themselves or with animals is as old as recorded human history. In Greek mythology, characters with the physical attributes of other creatures abound. Some were animals, such as Pegasus the winged horse or the Chimaera, which had a lion's head, a goat's body, and a serpent for a tail. Others were human in nature. The three Gorgons were fearsome female monsters with wings and writhing snakes for hair, and their visages could turn a person to stone. Even the mythic gods were not immune. The playful spirit Pan was a Satyr with horns, a goat's tail, and hooves for feet.

Although these ancient myths were the products of human imagination, evidence suggests that the foundation for transplantation began far before any other type of medical science was established. Archeological digs in France have established that surgery on the human body may have been one of the earliest medical accomplishments. Archeologists were astounded when they discovered the remains of human skulls that had undergone brain surgeries as far back as the Neolithic period, or Stone

Age. Furthermore, scientists ascertained that these surgeries were successful in that it appeared that the surgeries had taken place years prior to the people's deaths and were not the cause of those deaths. Brain surgery was also a therapy used extensively in the Americas by pre-Incan civilizations around 2,000 BC for a variety of problems, including mental illness, epilepsy, headaches, and head injuries.

One of the reasons for the early advancement of surgery was the warlike nature of society. Soldiers were routinely injured and maimed in battle, and the ancient healers sought to help them in any way possible. One of the earliest reports of an actual attempt at transplantation comes from an ancient Chinese text by Lieh Tsu, a Taoist sage who lived around 350 BC.

According to Tsu's account, the noted Chinese physician Pien Ch'iao (c. 500 BC) had cured two soldiers of an unidentified illness but told them that they also suffered from a congenital disease that caused one to have strong mental powers but a weak will, making the soldier strong in mental planning but unable to make decisions. He told the other soldier that he suffered from the opposite traits, leading this particular warrior to have strong willpower but a lack of forethought. Pien Ch'iao, who believed the heart to be the center of people's mental faculties, proposed to exchange the two soldiers' hearts as a cure that would establish equilibrium in their energies and mental powers. The soldiers agreed, and the doctor administered a strong potion of medicated wine to throw them into a death-like trance (which indicates that early physicians had at least the concept of anesthetics). He then opened their chest cavities and switched hearts and closed the wounds with a poultice of herbs. Although the text's statement that both men lived is dubious at best, this surgery is the first known medical account, whether real or legend, of the actual transfer of body organs between humans.

Over the centuries, the "idea" of transplantation for the most part remained immersed in religious beliefs and the supernatural. For example, Saint Mark in the first century AD was reported to have reattached the hand of a soldier after the soldier had lost the hand in battle. The brothers and Christian physicians Saint Cosmos and Saint Damian are considered the patron saints of transplantation for their reported miraculous replacement of the amputated leg of a Roman with that of a dark-skinned Ethiopian gladiator. The feat, which has been depicted in numerous paintings, is even more miraculous in its conception in that the two saints had been martyred by beheading years earlier and reappeared after death to perform the surgery.

Although such accounts of transplantation fall in the realm of legends and fantasy, believable reports of surgical reconstruction of the nose by grafting skin flaps date back to somewhere between 800 and 400 BC in ancient India, as reported by the Indian surgeon Susrata (or Sushruta) in his treatise *Susrata Samhita* (or *Sushruta Samhita*). This operation developed because of war injuries and the common punishment of cutting off noses, which led people to seek cosmetic remedy.

Unfortunately, because of social, religious, and cultural beliefs held by Arabs and later by Europeans, all types of surgery fell into disfavor and languished, eventually being taken over by the likes of barbers and bathkeepers. When surgery was once again established as a viable therapy during the Renaissance (c. 1400–1700), a renewed interest developed in skin grafting as operating skills and conditions somewhat improved.

In the sixteenth century, for example, Gaspare Tagliacozzi (sometimes spelled Tagliocozzi), who is considered the father of modern plastic surgery, transplanted the skin from patients' own arms to recreate whole noses for them and to repair damaged ears. In the 1740s, a French doctor named Garengeot reported that he grafted a soldier's nose back on using skin from another part of the soldier's body. Although these autografts (tissue taken from one site and grafted to another site on the same person) were generally successful, Tagliacozzi recognized early on that individual differences prevented tissue from being successfully transplanted between two individuals, now known as allografts (tissue or organ transplanted from a donor of the same species but different genetic makeup). In his treatise *De Curtorum Chirurgia per Insitionem* (1597), Tagliacozzi noted, "The singular character of the individual entirely dissuades us from attempting this work on another person. For such is the force and power of individuality, that if any one should believe that he could achieve even the least part of the operation, we consider him plainly superstitious and badly grounded in physical science."

ESTABLISHING THE FOUNDATION

Although scientists and medical researchers recognized early that innate differences in individuals prevented "swapping" skin and other body parts, scientific advances continued to be made that would ultimately lay the foundation for transplantation of organs between people. Blood transfusions, for example, began in earnest in the early 1800s in England. In Vienna in 1900, Karl Landsteiner discovered that blood serum from different individuals sometimes led to clumping of red blood cells in test tubes, which in turn led to the discovery of the major blood groups A, B, and O, which could then be matched to ensure safe transfusions. As Nicholas L. Tilney noted in his book *Transplant: From Myth to Reality*, "The obvious importance of matching donor serum and recipient cells before the administration of blood emphasized that, like skin-graft survival, individual differences between persons and between species limited indiscriminant transfer" (Tilney, 2003, p. 21).

Although medical science was making rapid advances at the beginning of the twentieth century, surgeons still faced many obstacles. Perhaps most daunting to surgeons at the time was their inability to quickly repair damaged arteries and veins. In 1894, French President Sadi Carnot was stabbed in the liver and his portal vein severed. The surgeons were essentially helpless as he bled to death in the hospital. A young French physician named Alexis Carrel realized that if the doctors could have repaired the portal vein, Carnot might have survived. As a result, Carnot developed successful techniques for sewing arteries and veins. He made his surgical advances by studying with some of the best embroiderers in France and by using extremely fine sutures made of silk, which allowed him to prevent clotting because of the silk thread's minimal impact on the smooth vascular lining. Carrel received the 1912 Nobel Prize in Medicine for his surgical advances.

Although advanced research into transplantation did not begin to take place until the early twentieth century, doctors and scientists had begun to experiment with the idea of transplantation in the eighteenth century. In 1749, for example, the naturalist and physiologist Henri-Louis Duhamel du Monceau was able to transplant spurs removed from young chickens onto the comb of the same animal and onto other chickens. In addition, numerous studies in skin grafting between animals took place in the nineteenth century. Giuseppe Boronio successfully grafted skin from one sheep onto the back of another sheep. John Hunter in England experimented with transplanting organs from male chickens into female chickens. In Ireland, Samuel Bigger transplanted a full cornea into the blind eye of a pet gazelle.

W.G. Thompson experimented with dogs and cats, removing the frontal lobes from their brains and replacing them with allografts. Although no neural or brain activity resulted, the grafts did last for some time. Reporting on his research in the *New York Medical Journal*, Thompson made perhaps one of the most prescient understatements in medical history when he wrote, "I think the main fact of this experiment—namely, that brain tissue has sufficient vitality to survive for seven weeks the operation of transplantation without wholly losing its identity as brain substance— suggests an interesting field for further research, and I have no doubt that other experimenters will be rewarded by investigating it" (Thompson, 1890).

EARLY HUMAN EXPERIMENTS

Experiments in transplantation focusing on humans began to spring up around the world at the beginning of the twentieth century. In 1906 the Austrian ophthalmologist Edward Zim performed the first successful corneal transplant in a human. Subsequent procedures enjoyed such a good rate of success that within only a few years corneal transplants were part of standard medical treatments for certain ailments that caused blindness. The reason for this early transplantation success is that corneas are not vascularized (that is, they do not have vessels to conduct and circulate fluids from other parts of the body), thus eliminating rejection problems associated with vascularized organs, which are directly connected to the blood and lymphatic system that cause immune responses to reject organs.

Research into transplantation continued with various bone, joint, and vascular transplants, all with widely varying outcomes. Carrel's advances in suturing techniques led to many experiments, mostly in France and Ukraine, that focused on transplanted pig and goat kidneys into dying humans as a last-ditch effort to save the human patients. Carrel also conducted transplantation experiments for several years in animals. Although he demonstrated early cold-storage techniques for preserving organs removed from the body, he eventually left the field when his long-term results showed that transplants between different animals of the same species were not viable. In 1906 Carrel's former teacher in France, Mathieu Jaboulay, made an early attempt at a kidney (renal) transplantation between humans. In an effort to try and assist urine excretion in two dying patients, Jaboulay grafted donor kidneys to their arm vessels, but the kidneys failed.

World War I and its burdens on the medical community distracted researchers from efforts in transplantation. In the years following the war, only a few doctors and scientists involved themselves in the field because it was apparent that some biological mechanisms were preventing acceptance of transplanted organs. Those who continued to study transplantation rarely committed their entire efforts to the endeavor. Their research focused on particular aspects of the field, such as organ preservation, drugs to increase urine flow in transplanted kidneys in animals, and genetic differences in dogs that caused organ rejection.

Only a few attempts at human transplantation occurred between World War I and World War II. In 1913 a young German girl with extreme inflammation of kidneys (nephritis) caused by mercury poisoning received a transplanted kidney taken from a Japanese monkey, which scientists had recently discovered shared similar red blood cell antigens (a substance that stimulates the production of antibodies) with humans.

Although the organ produced a small amount of urine, the girl died within three days of the transplant. In the United States, a similar procedure was attempted in 1923 for another patient suffering from mercury poisoning when Harold Neuhof transplanted a lamb's kidney into the patient, who died within nine days.

Yu Yu Voronoy of Russia conducted the most ardent transplantation research efforts in humans during this period. Voronoy, who had once studied using cadaver blood for transfusions, carried out a series of human-to-human renal transplants. During the 1930s, he took the kidneys from cadavers and transplanted them into six patients poisoned by chloride of mercury. None of the patients survived. Nevertheless, Voronoy, through his earlier work with dogs, is believed to have been the first researcher to detect specific serum antibodies in graft recipients that led to graft rejection.

FIRST SUCCESSFUL HUMAN ORGAN TRANSPLANT

Despite the universal failure to successfully transplant organs in humans, clinical advances in surgery and patient care along with new understanding of human biology spurred another generation of physician-scientists to reconsider transplantation as a potential treatment for people with end-stage organ failure. For the most part, researchers focused on the kidney, largely because it was a relatively "convenient" organ to access and surgically transplant. Scientists had also revealed a great deal about its physiology and the relationship between some diseases and kidney pathology, that is, its variation from a healthy or normal condition.

In 1947 three surgeons at the Peter Bent Brigham Hospital in Boston—Ernest Landsteiner, Charles Hufnagel, and David Hume—sought to save the life of a young woman dying from acute renal failure resulting from a septic abortion and hemorrhage. The doctors felt that if the patient could survive the immediate danger—or acute episode—of kidney failure, the kidney would regain its function. However, they needed a healthy kidney to temporarily do the work of the woman's failing kidney. A hospital employee agreed to donate the kidney of a relative who had just died, and the surgeons connected the kidney to the woman via a major artery and vein in the patient's elbow. Although the woman's kidney recovered and began to function normally, she eventually died from hepatitis, which she had contracted from an earlier blood transfusion.

Another example of using a cadaver kidney as a "temporary bridge" until the native kidney could begin to function occurred in 1950 in Chicago. Richard Lawler took a kidney from a patient who had just died from liver disease and connected it to another patient's renal vessels. The patient, Ruth Tucker, had a blood type similar to the donor, and the new kidney worked, emitting urine and continuing to function after fifty-three days. Although ten months later the transplanted kidney was no longer functioning, the patient continued to live for five more years. In essence, the operation succeeded because it had allowed the patient's own kidney enough time to recover and resume at least partial functioning.

Although there were some early concerns and censures from others in the medical field, these positive results spurred new interest in transplantation. The belief that perhaps transplantation could work with kidneys was also bolstered by the development of dialysis, which could be used to help support the patient if the kidney failed. Hume, who had helped foster the interest in kidney transplantation in Boston, went on to conduct nine kidney transplants in patients using cadaver kidneys and a less invasive approach similar to the methods used by Voronoy in his unsuccessful attempts in the 1930s. Hume's approach involved connecting the renal artery and the vein from the donated kidney to the vessels in the patients' groins. He then covered the kidney with a skin flap from the upper thigh. Although the first eight patients died shortly after the transplant, the ninth recipient survived for five-and-a-half months before succumbing to kidney failure. Hume and others explained this extended survival time as being related to unidentified similarities that must have existed between the donor and host.

Despite some initial promising results, enthusiasm began to fade as patients invariably died because the transplanted kidneys only functioned temporarily. In general, the patients seemed overly susceptible to infections. Furthermore, the patient's immune system inevitably destroyed the transplanted kidneys, or grafts. These failures led to a growing consensus that transplant surgery would never succeed.

THE HERRICKS

The floundering field of transplantation received a significant booster shot on December 23, 1954, when Boston surgeon Joseph E. Murray performed the first successful transplant of an organ from one human to another. Murray removed a kidney from Ronald Herrick and implanted it into his identical twin brother Richard, the victim of a fatal kidney disease. Murray had been doing experiments with allografts in dogs and knew, along with many of his colleagues, that skin grafts between identical twins had been shown to survive indefinitely in several cases. As a result, Murray and his group at Peter Bent Brigham Hospital immediately thought of a transplant when they learned that Richard Herrick had a twin

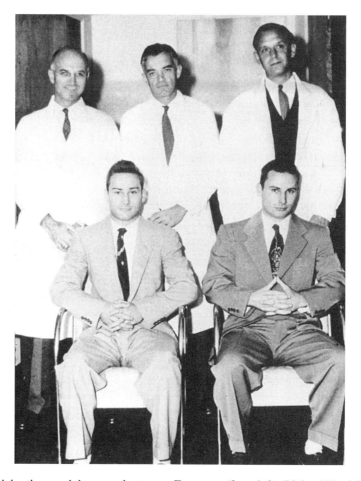

Herrick brothers and the transplant team. Front row (from left): Richard Herrick, kidney transplant recipient; Ronald Herrick, kidney donor. Back row (from left): Brigham transplant team—Joseph E. Murray, M.D., surgeon for the recipient; John P. Merrill, M.D., nephrologist and co-leader of the team; J. Hartwell Harrison, M.D., urological surgeon for the donor. (Photograph courtesy of Brigham and Women's Hospital.)

brother. Before the transplant, the doctors confirmed that the brothers had shared a common placenta and all known blood groups. They even went so far as take the brother's fingerprints and have them examined at the local police station, where they proved to be identical.

Once Murray and his colleagues revascularized the kidney after transplantation, the organ produced urine immediately. Richard recovered quickly and went on to live nine more years until he died of a heart attack.

Prior to this breakthrough, transplantation had numerous critics who were blatantly unenthusiastic about the therapy's potential and sometimes downright derisive. "We were told it was impossible and that we were playing God and shouldn't do it," said Murray on the National Kidney Foundation Web site honoring transplantation's fiftieth anniversary (National Kidney Foundation, 2005). In 1990 Murray shared the Nobel Prize in Physiology or Medicine for his achievement.

More successful kidney transplants among identical twins took place over the next two decades at Brigham and elsewhere, including Montreal and Paris. Among the twin recipients were women who became pregnant and had babies, as well as children whose renal failure had stunted their growth but who grew rapidly after their successful transplants. It was the first real proof that end-stage organ disease could be turned around through transplantation and that patients could be brought back from the brink of death to go on and lead normal lives.

OVERCOMING THE IMMUNE BARRIER

Despite the success with twins, those pioneering the field of transplantation knew that they had some major obstacles to overcome before transplantation could be considered a viable therapy. Although a few clinical observations had been made concerning grafts and rejection prior to World War II, it was Peter Medawar, a young English zoologist, who began to place the study of immunology on a solid scientific basis. Working with a plastic surgeon named Thomas Gibson during World War II, Medawar noticed an interesting phenomenon. Not only were skin grafts from donors ultimately destroyed on patients, but, additionally, a second graft from the same donor was destroyed even more quickly than the first graft. Medawar's conclusion was that rejection "was brought about by a mechanism of active immunization" and that the process included "memory," which enabled the body's immunization process to work even faster when it encountered the same foreign invader again.

Medawar continued his studies of foreign-tissue rejection in rabbits and started to unravel the changes associated with rejection as initiated by a genetically dissimilar host. Others soon joined Medawar in the 1950s in trying to understand and break down the immune barrier that was the major obstacle to transplantation. Medawar and colleagues showed that lymphocytes (a type of white blood cell) in a skin transplant recipient gathered in large numbers in the skin grafts prior to destruction of the tissue. As a result, a great deal of research began to focus on these cells.

By the early 1950s, researchers had confirmed that lymphocytes initiate an immune response through interaction with antigens, which are substances such as enzymes or toxins that stimulate the production of antibodies. Working at Oxford in England in the 1960s, James Gowans revealed that many lymphocytes circulate continuously in tissues, lymph, and blood. Gowans also showed that these cells' ability to reject stable skin grafts meant that they were "immunologically competent." Another Oxford scientist, Rodney Porter, and Gerald Edelman, who was working in New York, brought about a greater understanding of antibodies produced by lymphocytes and the role they played in immunity when both scientists independently defined the structure of immunoglobulin (a class of proteins produced in lymph tissue).

While these advances in the study of immunology were being made, surgeons continued their efforts to expand the boundaries of transplantation. By 1960, experimental transplantation models for all the major organs had been established in animals. In 1963 Starzl, then at the University of Colorado, performed the first human liver transplant. In that same year, James Hardy of the University of Mississippi completed the first lung transplant. Christiaan Barnard performed the first heart transplant in 1967 in South Africa. For the most part, however, results were dismal because the immune barrier proved too strong. Starzl, for example, was so distressed by the results of his liver transplants that he placed a moratorium on performing any more transplants until advances could be made in overcoming rejection problems.

Early experiments to suppress the immune system focused on using total-body X-radiation in animals. By the late 1950s, several patients in Boston and Paris had undergone this treatment before receiving a kidney from a cadaver. All but two died quickly, but one patient from Boston survived and then lived for twenty more years without receiving any other immunosuppression, and a patient in Paris lived for twenty-six years. The cause of death for both was unrelated to their transplant. Nevertheless, total-body X-radiation had several drawbacks, including unreliability and serious side effects that often proved fatal.

In 1959 Robert Schwarts and Walter Dameshek of Tufts University discovered the first drugs that could suppress immune responses. They found that an anti-metabolite, 6-mercaptopurine (6-MP), inhibited the formation of antibodies in rabbits. Roy Calne in England and Charles Zukoski at the University of Virginia quickly followed up on this discovery and showed independently that this agent increased kidney graft survival in dogs. Meanwhile, during the moratorium on liver transplants, Starzl and colleagues began making advances that would prove applicable to all organ

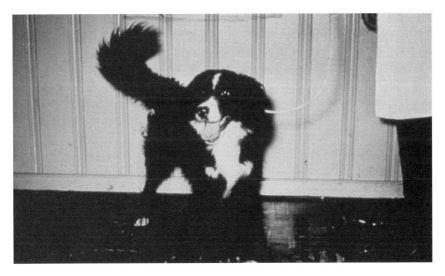

Starzl conducted liver transplantation studies in dogs during a three-and-a-half-year voluntary moratorium on liver transplantation in the mid-1960s. Studies with these animals resulted in many long-surviving recipients, including this one that lived for thirteen years. The animals were treated with a short course of immunosuppressive drugs. (Photo courtesy of Dr. Starzl.)

transplants. The most important area of advancement was the improvement of immunosuppression. In experiments with dogs, Starzl and colleagues showed that a preparation of antilymphocyte globulin (ALG) in combination with the drugs Imuran and prednisone resulted in extended survival, with one dog ultimately living for thirteen years after receiving a liver transplant.

With the field buoyed by the results of this discovery, the moratorium on liver transplantation was rescinded in 1967. Although less than half of the transplants succeeded in the initial cases, the ones that were successful had a domino effect, leading to the first successful human heart, pancreas, and lung transplants, all of which used the Denver triple-drug immunosuppression. A beachhead for clinical transplantation was finally established.

A VIABLE THERAPY

The initial, albeit tenuous, successes in overcoming the immune system in the 1960s led to a groundswell of interest in a field that was beginning to achieve a sense of legitimacy. Young researchers were drawn to the field by the notion that new discoveries, innovations, and advances were not only possible but even probable. Nevertheless, patient mortality remained high, and long-term graft survival was unsatisfactory. Even in kidney transplants, which had been explored the most extensively in terms of research and the number of transplants performed, graft function at one year for cadaver donor grafts was only 45 percent. Nonidentical, living-related donor kidneys, however, fared much better with a 70 percent survival rate. Even in the first decade of kidney transplants between 1954 and 1964, U.S. surgeons performed more than 600 transplants between living persons (not necessarily related), achieving a two-year survival rate of around 50 percent. Still, kidney and other transplant patients suffered from the continuous maintenance immunosuppression that they received, causing many to die of opportunistic infections by fungi and viruses that their suppressed immune systems could not battle successfully. Many transplant recipients also developed cancer. Other serious side effects included obesity, easily damaged skin, and bone death and fractures.

Despite its potential to save lives, transplantation still had far to go to reach full legitimacy. Another major breakthrough occurred in 1979 when Calne and colleagues at Cambridge reported on the use of the immunosuppressive drug cyclosporine A. In their report, published in the November 1978 issue of *Lancet*, the researchers noted that twenty-six of thirty-two transplanted kidneys effectively functioned without rejection, as well as two pancreases and two livers. In addition, no other steroids were used in twenty patients, and no additional immunosuppression was given to fifteen patients, thus cutting back on the incident of side effects for these drugs. The new treatment approach with cyclosporine led to a rapid growth in transplantation in the 1980s when numerous advances were made in the field. In the 1990s, the development of the drug FK-506 (tacrolimus), largely under the guidance of Starzl, who had moved to the University of Pittsburgh, further increased the effectiveness of transplantation. These new successes resulted in a dramatic growth in the field, both in terms of surgeons and other specialists focusing their efforts on transplantation and in the spread of transplant centers throughout the United States and the world.

At the end of 2001, data analyses of 110,000 renal transplants in the United States performed over the previous ten years showed that cadaver kidney grafts had achieved functional survival rates of approximately 90 percent at one year, 80 percent over three years, and 40 percent at ten years. The rates from living donors were even better. In a review of 40,000 liver transplants performed over that same time period, adult recipients had an 86 percent survival rate at one year and a 76 percent survival rate at three years. Other types of organ transplants also showed vast improvement in survival rates, such as heart transplants, with about 85 percent of recipients surviving at one year and 77 percent at five years.

Since Richard Herrick received a kidney from his brother Ronald, more than 400,000 transplants have been performed. Today, few would argue that transplantation has not evolved into a viable therapy for a host of serious conditions and diseases. By the dawn of the twenty-first century, transplantation had become a firmly established therapy that offered new hope for approximately 40,000 patients each year throughout the world.

The future of transplantation lies in many areas and is moving beyond just the transplantation of organs and tissues. The transplantation of cells and genes, for example, is under investigation for both curing and preventing diseases, such as Parkinson's disease, muscular dystrophy, and spinal cord injuries. Liver cell transplants may one day help cure deadly metabolic disease or prevent the need for a liver organ transplant. Islet cells are another area that shows promise for treating diabetes. In Type 1 diabetes, the immune system destroys the islet cells needed for producing insulin. In islet cell transplantation, the destroyed insulin-producing cells are replaced with functioning donor cells recovered from the pancreas of recently deceased donors. Another area of research, although highly controversial, is embryonic, or fetal, cell transplants for the treatment of neurological disorders such as Parkinson's disease and Huntingdon's disease (see Chapter 9).

One of the major obstacles to transplantation for many patients is the lack of donor organs. As a result, research into cross-species transplantation (xenotransplantation) is underway. For example, researchers at the Thomas E. Starzl Transplantation Institute are studying the possibility of using organs from genetically modified pigs. A significant area of research also focuses on the development of artificial organs, most notably the artificial heart.

Finally, although transplantation has come a long way in providing more effective and safer immunosuppression protocols for transplant patients, more work has to be done. A new area of research focuses on the possibility of weaning patients completely off of immunosuppressant drugs, which still have many serious side effects. In addition to affecting the patients themselves, these drugs may affect a female transplant recipient's offspring. According to several studies, women who have received a transplant and are taking immunosuppressive drugs have a high rate of childbirth complications, with up to half of the women having small, preterm babies. Furthermore, approximately 30 percent of the babies develop hypertension, and another 30 percent have infections. There is also concern over these babies' future in terms of neurocognitive problems such as learning. These children may also have a high incidence of autoimmune disorders, in which the individual's immune system mistakenly attacks the individual's own tissues.

By 2004, the year that marked the fiftieth anniversary of the first successful human organ transplant, new efforts were underway in transplanting limbs and appendages. For example, surgeons have now performed hand transplants with varying degrees of success. Several groups of transplant surgeons also have announced that they are pursuing the transplantation of faces, and "partial" face transplants have already been performed in France and China. Through years of animal research, scientists now can excise an entire face from a brain-dead body, including nose cartilage, nerves, and muscles. The idea is to suture the excised face to the hairline and jaw of someone whose face has been grotesquely disfigured. An ethical debate has arisen about the procedure, focusing on a series of complex ethical questions, including the long-term safety of such transplants because of the need for higher immunosuppressive therapy, the uncertain outcome in terms of normal looks and functioning, and the emotional impact on the recipient who will no longer physically appear to be the same person.

But controversy in transplantation is not new. As Starzl noted in a 2003 speech to a gathering of transplant professionals in Germany and as quoted in the Thomas E. Starzl Transplantation Newsletter *MATCH* (Spring 2005), "Every major advance in liver and other kinds of organ transplantation of the last half century has required the overthrow of some scientific dogma or the revision of a social, ethical, or legal doctrine. Consequently, the ascension of transplantation was more a fifty-year war against the status quo, than an orderly evolution" (Petechuk, 2005, p. 3).

CONTROVERSY FROM THE BEGINNING

What Starzl describes as a "war" began with the very first successful human transplant involving the Herrick brothers. In essence, the ethical dilemma in this case stemmed from one of the oldest and most well-known imperatives in medicine, namely, "First, do no harm." Although attributed to Greek physician Hippocrates (460–377 BC), the phrase does not appear in the Hippocratic Oath that physicians take when entering medical practice. Nevertheless, most scholars of medical history believe that Hippocrates did originate the phrase in his writings *Epidemics*. Others trace the origins to an earlier Latin source and the phrase, "Primum

An Early Scandal

Although modern drugs have been developed to treat impotence (also known as erectile dysfunction) in men, the search for reinvigorating the male's sexual drive and performance is ancient. For example, the Chinese used rhinoceros horns for thousands of years as an aphrodisiac, and another Asian remedy was a soup made from boiled mussels. In the United States in the 1920s, new knowledge about the endocrine glands and the successful use of endocrine-based products such as insulin for diabetes led to research into the transplantation of testes. In the early 1900s, Sergei Voronoff had begun conducting experiments in Paris in which he transplanted slices of monkey testes into nearly a thousand patients. Some went on to claim that the transplants had reinvigorated them. The idea grew in popularity despite the fact that no concrete scientific evidence proved that such transplants actually had any effect. Even the *Boston Medical and Surgical Journal*, which would later become the *New England Journal of Medicine*, ruminated in an editorial that it was likely that the transplants had some effects.

While some began investigating the phenomenon, a charlatan in Milford, Kansas, named John Romulus Brinkley began inserting into men's testicles the glands of a virile goat. Brinkley had failed in his attempts to get into medical school but nevertheless set up a practice in the small Kansas town. He had read about Voronoff, but because he did not have access to monkeys, he used goats based on their reputation as lusty animals. When one of Brinkley's first patients commented that he believed his sex life had improved and he then impregnated his wife, Brinkley's transplant practice soared. Men sometimes paid up to $750 for the operation, a significant sum in the 1920s. When Brinkley was forced to stop practicing medicine by the Kansas State Board of Medicine, he hired licensed physicians to perform the operation for him.

Eventually, scientific data from research began to emerge showing that testicular transplantation was not effective, and common sense eventually prevailed. As for Brinkley, he had made a fortune that enabled him to buy a radio station and run for governor, a race that he narrowly lost. Following a number of lawsuits, including some by former patients who had experienced adverse side effects from the operations, he was forced to declare bankruptcy by 1941.

non nocere," which appears in the later writings of the Roman physician, Galen (131–201 AD).

Regardless of the phrase's origins, it has been accepted as a basic tenant in the practice of medicine for approximately two thousand years. The question that first arose with Ronald Herrick's donation of a kidney to his brother was whether or not the removal of a functioning organ from a perfectly healthy individual was in fact a type of "harm." The operation did pose a serious risk to the donor. Furthermore, at that time, the potential benefit to the recipient was tenuous at best considering that surgeons had never successfully transplanted an organ into a human being.

Murray and his transplant team were well aware of this issue and appeared to make every effort to inform Ronald Herrick of the risks involved and did not urge him to undergo the donation surgery to save his brother's life. In their talks with Herrick, the team discussed a variety of ethical, philosophical, and medical issues designed to reinforce the donor's understanding that he had the freedom and moral right not to choose to donate a kidney to his brother. Herrick agreed to the transplant only after the surgical team promised to continue to address any medical problems he might have in the future that might arise from his donation.

The first court case focusing on the ethics of transplantation occurred in 1957, just three years after the successful transplant between the Herrick brothers, when a Massachusetts court began hearing the case of a proposed kidney transplantation between identical twins who were under legal age. Obviously, parental consent was needed for the operation, but the specter of performing an operation on a perfectly healthy child loomed over the proceedings. The court ultimately ruled in favor of allowing the operation as long as the parents and the healthy child consented. The court based its decision largely on the testimony of psychiatrists who said they believed that the healthy twin also benefited from the operation because the child might suffer psychologically in the future if the twin sibling died.

The idea that transplantation also promoted the future welfare of the donor was further strengthened in the courts in a 1969 Kentucky case. This time, however, the donor, Jerry Strunk, was not a minor but mentally disabled. The ethical questions arose because the donor could not be considered mentally competent to make the difficult decision of donating an organ and fully understand the risks involved. Once again, the court maneuvered around the "do no harm" maxim by deciding that the donor would ultimately benefit from the operation because he was devoted to his sick brother, whose death would have a negative impact on Jerry and whose life would ultimately prove to be a benefit to Jerry's well-being.

Several issues concerning transplantation were brought up in a 1964 article by Russell Elkington in the *Annals of Internal Medicine*. The ethical and moral problems addressed by Elkington included the idea that transplantation might fail to live up to expectations concerning health and the chances of long-term survival. He also noted that transplantation required the physicians to choose among patients, primarily because of the relatively few resources for donor organs, which also meant that the procedure applied to a relatively small patient population. Furthermore, Elkington was among the first to address the question of whether it was ethical or moral to focus so many medical and financial resources on a procedure that had uncertain outcomes. Elkington's article led to a significant response from many of those currently working to push the field forward. Although the general consensus among this small cadre of pioneering transplant specialists was that they had undergone a great deal of their own "soul searching" concerning the ethics of transplantation, they nevertheless stated that the field should not be abandoned because it would ultimately advance and one day give hope and life to many people.

In 1966 Sir Michael Woodruff, a British transplant specialist, collaborated with the CIBA Foundation to hold a meeting on the ethical and legal issues surrounding organ transplantation. Those attending the three-day meeting included doctors, lawyers, ethicists, and others. They raised a number of important issues, most of which continue to be debated and studied. For example, they wondered whether the medical community could ensure that a donor was not unduly influenced to make a donation. They asked, how can certain populations, such as children, prisoners, and the mentally handicapped, be protected from unwittingly being organ donors or participants in clinical research trials? They also discussed such issues as animal research, the law in relation to the essential mutilation of a donor for the advantage of someone else, and the extent that society must help support the costs for sustaining life through transplantation or other new medical advances and technologies.

The short meeting of these distinguished professionals did little to solve any of these issues, but it represented a significant step in acknowledging that the medical community and society in general would have to address these ethical dilemmas. In 1967, less than a year after the meeting, which produced the publication *Law and Ethics of Transplantation*, a new ethical issue surrounding transplantation quickly arose. Christiaan Barnard performed a heart transplant at the Groote Schuur Hospital in Cape Town, South Africa. What spurred the public's interest and concern beyond the idea of potentially achieving success in transplanting a human heart was the question of where Barnard had obtained the donor organ. He had, in fact, retrieved the still-beating heart from a twenty-two-year-old woman named Denise Daarvall, who had suffered irreversible brain damage in a car accident the day before.

The patient who received Daarvall's heart, Louis Washkansky, was suffering from terminal heart disease. Although he lived for only eighteen days following the transplant, the operation was publicized worldwide and initiated a surge in both professional and public interest in the ethics of transplantation. Foremost in people's minds was the idea of brain death: just exactly when could or should a person be classified as being dead? It became apparent that all patients who were comatose were now essentially "targets" for having their organs removed. This idea, in turn, raised for the first time questions about how much doctors should be trusted to make such decisions as well as whether or not comatose patients should even be used at all for procuring organs.

As a result of Banard's operation, an ad hoc committee was formed at Harvard Medical School to try to develop a definition of "irreversible coma." The committee included a wide range of professionals, from a variety of medical specialists, including a psychiatrist, to a lawyer and a theologian. In a 1968 article published in the *Journal of the American Medical Association*, the committee concluded that it could be agreed upon medically and morally that after a certain time "it is no longer appropriate to continue extraordinary means of support for the hopelessly unconscious patient." Furthermore, the committee stated that "a strong case can be made that society can ill afford to discard the tissues and organs of hopelessly unconscious patients so greatly needed for study and experimental trials to help those who can be salvaged" (Ad Hoc Committee of the Harvard Medical School to Examine the Definition of Brain Death, 1968). The committee went on to comment that the donation, however, must be made with the approval of the family involved and had to be sanctioned by law. Of course, this was only the beginning of the debate.

The committee's efforts could not have come any sooner. Legal problems were arising surrounding the acquisition of donor hearts. In Richmond, Virginia, heart transplant surgeon Richard Lower went on trial for murder because he used a heart from someone dying from a severe brain injury. The trial marked the first time a jury was instructed to consider a legal definition of the end of life as being associated with brain death. Lower was eventually acquitted of the charge. Another scandal in Japan in the late 1960s was similar to the Lower case. It was so detrimental to the Japanese public's view of heart transplantation that another heart transplant was not performed in that country for approximately three decades.

Although *Time* magazine deemed 1969 "The Year of the Transplant," the outcomes of continuing heart transplants by Banard and others were not encouraging, despite the fact that Banard's second heart transplant patient, Philip Blaiberg, lived for 594 days. By June of 1970, only ten recipients out of the 142 who had received transplants in the prior two-and-a-half years or so were still alive. After *Life* magazine wrote a story about the "heart transplant tragedy," the "Miracle of Capetown" was seen in an increasingly negative light by the public and the government, both of which began to question whether such operations should be performed. By the mid-1970s, an unofficial moratorium on heart transplants was in effect.

The field of transplantation only faced more questions as it progressed and became more successful in the 1980s. Questions about organ allocation increased, and the issue of supply and demand came to the forefront as more and more patients began to seek an increasingly effective treatment for end-stage organ diseases. With such a scarce resource, priority issues inevitably surfaced. For example, should alcoholics receive liver transplants, given that they destroyed their livers through their own negligence? Should prison inmates be chosen to receive an organ over a law-abiding citizen? Should selection be random or based on some type of criteria? Furthermore, as the costs of health care began to rise dramatically, many questioned the ethics of a society investing a scarce resource in what still appeared to be a relatively limited "return" on investment not only in terms of saving lives but also in terms of the actual number of years the transplant recipient would live.

Most of these ethical and moral issues remain in debate. For example, despite the success of living-donor organ transplants, a few donor patients have died in the process, leading to the continuation of the ethical and moral questions about harming a healthy person. New issues are also arising. The chance that transplantation between species, called xenotransplantation, may be possible has opened up a series of ethical issues concerning the spread of disease, animal rights, and judicious use of resources.

Another growing debate is the ethics and plausibility of offering financial incentives for organ donation. The limited supply of organs has also led to potential abuses in using organs unfit for transplantation and in lowering the standards for determining the donor organs deemed acceptable for transplantation. Already, kidney transplant candidates can sign up for an extended donor list that would allow donor kidneys to be used under a less stringent criteria and would include kidneys from donors over sixty and donors over fifty who have risk factors for damaged kidneys. Ethicists are also concerned about full disclosure to patients over increased risks and allowing the patients to make their own decisions regarding whether to accept an extended-criteria kidney. Nevertheless, the shortage of donor organs is so great that extended criteria are being looked into for the transplantation of liver, heart, and lungs.

CHAPTER 2

Organ Procurement: Supply and Demand

Although during transplantation's infancy only a few visionaries saw the therapy's full potential, by the dawn of the twenty-first century, the field's phenomenal success could not be denied. In 2004 a total of 27,036 organ transplants were performed in the United States alone. Furthermore, by the year 2000, one-year survival rates had reached between 76 and 94 percent for recipients of heart, liver, pancreas, and kidney transplants. Quality of life for transplant patients has also improved. In their book *The U.S. Organ Procurement System: A Prescription for Reform*, David L. Kaserman and A. H. Barnett noted that "unlike many new medical technologies that tend to prolong a patient's life without significantly improving the quality of that life, organ transplantation often restores the patient's health to a level approximating that experienced before the onset of the disease" (Kaserman and Barnett, 2002, p. 2).

Perhaps most indicative of organ transplantation's ability to offer new life and hope is that patients are lining up for an opportunity to get a transplant. The bad news is that organs are in limited supply. As of late 2005, 90,249 people were on the organ transplant waiting list, but between January and the end of August that same year, only 9,795 organs had been donated. The concept of "supply and demand" is a driving market force in business, but it raises serious dilemmas and ethical questions in the field of transplantation. Simply put, there are not enough organs for all who need them, which has resulted in a life-or-death scenario for thousands of patients. How serious is the problem? In 2004 a new name was added to the organ transplant waiting list approximately every thirteen minutes, and each day an average of seventeen people died while waiting for a lifesaving organ that never came.

The basic problem is twofold. First, since the early days of success, the field of transplantation has faced the dilemma of obtaining enough lifesaving organs. Organ donation has always lagged behind the need, and early on, the medical community, along with the federal and state governments, began working to establish an ethical and effective procurement system. The system in place has worked well up to a point. Nevertheless, many argue that its failure to keep supply in pace with demand clearly shows that a new approach is needed to resolve the issue of providing organs for all those who need them. Some have proposed that the current system based on the notion of altruism and volunteerism should be abandoned for a market-based approach to the problem. Others are focusing on alternate sources of donor tissues and organs, such as organs from pigs and other animals.

One thing is clear. The failure to meet demand has led to the second dilemma concerning the allocation of organs. Because not enough organs are available, patients must be carefully selected to ensure the most effective use of a limited resource. Choosing one patient over another is, as the British would say, a "sticky wicket." Who decides who gets an organ? What are the basic criteria? Should patients be chosen because of need, likelihood of successful outcome, or a combination of both? Should some people be denied a transplant, such as alcoholics whose drinking caused their liver cirrhosis? Is it fair to allocate a donated resource more often to someone who has money or can afford insurance as opposed to others who may be less fortunate?

These and other ethical questions are addressed in subsequent chapters. First, this chapter relates how the current procurement system was established and operates, and the next chapter delves into the issue of allocation.

BRAIN DEATH

The rudimentary but incomplete answer to the problems of where and how to obtain organs lies with the concept of brain death. Although some organs, such as kidneys and livers, can be obtained through living donors, as in the way Richard Herrick received a kidney from his twin brother Ronald, the vast majority of organs come from organ donors who have died, referred to in the medical community as "cadaveric donors" and "cadaveric transplants." The concept of "brain death" is fundamental to organ donation for several reasons. Once a person dies, oxygen stops circulating through the blood stream, and the body's tissues and internal organs rapidly deteriorate, making them unsuitable for transplantation. For a transplanted organ to function properly, organ donors must have healthy and well-functioning organs. Organ donors must also be free of infections and have no cancer because the immunosuppressive drugs used in transplantation tend to accelerate the spread of cancer, or metastasis. As a result of these criteria, most organ donors come from people who are declared "brain dead" as a result of an accidental head injury or a stroke.

Prior to the 1950s, before medical technology was developed that could keep people alive on ventilators, or breathing machines, the common-law definition of death declared that a person was dead when his or her heart stopped beating, causing complete stoppage of blood circulation and the end of vital functions. This definition soon became problematic because of ventilators and the development of cardiopulmonary resuscitation (CPR), which could restore cardiopulmonary functioning but not necessarily brain function. Deprived of oxygen for too long, the brain can no longer function. Nevertheless, patients can be kept alive indefinitely on a ventilator, even though there is no hope for recovery.

The growing interest in the then fledgling but promising field of transplantation in the 1950s and 1960s led many to recognize that substantial criteria had to be established for brain death. When Christiaan Barnard obtained a donor heart in 1967 from a woman with an irreversible head injury, the issue of organ donation and procurement loomed as a dilemma that could halt transplantation in its tracks. As noted by Nicholas L. Tilney in *Transplant: From Myth to Reality*, "Indeed beneath all the enthusiasm and media frenzy concerning Barnard's operation lay public skepticism about the ethics of the procedure, mistrust of the autonomy of the medical profession, doubt about the use of patients in irreversible coma as donors, and even more primitive fears of premature burial" (Tilney, 2003, p.161).

As a result of these developments, a decision was made to establish the Ad Hoc Committee of the Harvard Medical School to Examine the Definition of Brain Death. In their 1968 landmark report, the committee laid out a set of criteria for determining brain death, with the major criteria essentially stating that death of the entire brain means that the person is dead. The committee stated that the brain was dead when it was no longer receiving blood and the essential oxygen that it carries for physical functioning. Such a definition was crucial for obtaining organs from donors because the rest of the body could still function normally and maintain healthy, functioning organs.

The American Medical Association (AMA) followed up on the Harvard committee's definition in 1974 by recognizing brain death as one of the suitable criteria for establishing the diagnosis of death. The AMA's recognition further established the basis for legal criteria concerning the recognition and diagnosis of brain death. The following year, the American Bar Association (ABA) House of Delegates developed the following definition of death: "For all legal purposes, a human body with irreversible

Brain Death and the Japanese

Different cultures struggle with issues of life and death in various ways. As a result, the issue of brain death and organ donation has faced resistance in some countries. Although the logical suspicion is that the problem would be more profound in nonindustrialized cultures, the technologically advanced Japanese have long struggled with the issue. In 1968 a Japanese surgeon, Toshiro Wada, performed the world's second heart transplant using a brain-dead donor organ. Before long, Wada found himself arrested for murder and entangled in a six-year court battle.

Although Wada was acquitted, the term "heart transplantation" was virtually forbidden within the Japanese culture for the next decade, despite the fact that nearly 50 percent of Japanese people said they equated brain death with final human death. By the beginning of the 1980s, however, Japanese society was conducting an intense debate over the issue, a debate that would last for the next fifteen years. In addition to the Wada case, many observers felt that a number of factors hindered Japanese acceptance of brain death for obtaining organs. For example, some Japanese still adhere to a traditional view that the body and soul remain together and are reunited in the next life. Other noted problems included physician mistrust and serious concerns over the criteria to establish brain death.

In 1997 Japan's Organ Transplantation Law was finally passed. Although it established criteria for brain death and the rights of individual Japanese citizens to declare their wishes to be organ donors, the law still enabled families to refuse the donation of their loved ones' organs. It took a year-and-a-half after the Japanese law's passage before surgeons performed the first "legal" heart, cornea, kidney, and liver transplant procedures using organs from a brain-dead donor.

Unlike most industrialized nations, Japan still remains relatively unique in its emphasis on living donor organs. A 1999 U.S. report stated that approximately 70 percent of transplanted kidneys and 80 percent of segmental liver procedures performed in Japan had come from live donors, whereas in the United States 68 percent of kidneys and 98 percent of livers transplanted in 1998 were obtained from cadaveric donors. According to the Japan Organ Transplant Network, in 2005 approximately thirty-eight brain-dead donors, or 6 percent, had been used for transplantation since the passage of the 1997 law. More than half of potentially brain-dead donors were not used because hospitals were not equipped to determine brain death or because relatives objected.

cessation of total brain function, according to usual and customary standards of medical practice, shall be considered dead" ("Guidelines for the Determination of Death," 1981). It is important to note that because of technology such as the electroencephalogram (EEG), physicians can determine whether the brain has ceased electrical activity, which is known as "cerebral silence." Diagnosis of brain death is further enhanced by cerebral angiography, which enables doctors to easily determine if there is a complete absence of blood flow to the brain.

In 1980 the National Conference of Commissioners on the Uniform State Laws, a national body made up of lawyers and designed to provide states with nonpartisan and effective legislation to consider, laid out its recommendations for establishing brain death through the adoption of the Uniform Determination of Death Act (UDODA). The act states, "An individual who has sustained either (1) irreversible cessation of circulatory and respiratory functions, or (2) irreversible cessation of all functions of the entire brain, including the brainstem, is dead" ("Guidelines for the Determination of Death," 1981). These criteria were endorsed by the AMA and ABA and eventually accepted throughout the United States through legislation enacted by all fifty states.

PROCURING ORGANS

The Uniform Anatomical Gift Act of 1968

Although the establishment of brain death was the first lynchpin in the development of transplantation, the field's pioneers still faced the dilemma of acquiring appropriate organs in a timely and effective manner. Transplantation was already saving lives and leading to a serious debate among physicians and ethicists concerning cadaveric organ procurement. One of the key issues was how to make sure that individuals had the right to donate organs and tissues. Equally important in the estimation of those pondering these issues at that time, however, was the philosophy that organs should not be used without the permission of the individual or family under the concept of the donor's "presumed consent."

To encourage organ donation in the United States and to address some of the legal and ethical issues of transplantation, the National Conference of Commissioners on the Uniform State Laws and the American Bar Association approved the Uniform Anatomical Gift Act (UAGA) of 1968. In essence, the UAGA established the legal foundation for cadaveric organ donation while trying to address the issue of competing interests in organ donation and transplantation. At the same time, the act's aim was to ensure individual autonomy and dignity by preventing presumed consent legislation from being enacted.

The UAGA defined "competing interests" to include the wishes of the deceased and the deceased's relatives, the state's need to perform autopsies to determine the cause of death in a crime or in other circumstances, and society's need for tissues and organs (not only for transplantation but also for medical education and research). Placing these competing interests in a hierarchy, the UAGA recommended that the most respect be given to the individual's wishes made during his or her lifetime, as made clear in an organ donor card or will, if possible. Furthermore, the individual's wishes were also to be honored if a statement was made not to donate an organ, even if surviving relatives expressed the desire to make an organ donation. If the deceased did not make clear his or her wish to donate an organ, the UAGA prioritized the list of people who could authorize donation, beginning with the spouse and followed by adult children, parents, siblings, grandparents, and finally a legal guardian. If no family member could be found to make such a decision, the UAGA also authorized the local coroner, medical examiner, or public health officer to allow the removal of organs and tissues for transplantation. To provide other safeguards to help prevent conflicts of interest, the UAGA declared that the doctor who declares a patient dead and the doctor who removes the organ cannot be the same person.

The UAGA of 1968 was a significant first step in addressing the need for organs by developing a legal basis for an ethical nationwide system of organ procurement. Perhaps most important was UAGA's establishment of an individual's right to sign a document agreeing to have his or her organs donated. The UAGA categorically stated that once such a document had been signed, hospitals did not need to gain further permission from family to use the individual's organs. By 1973, every state had adopted the UAGA's recommendations in some version.

The National Organ Transplant Act

By the early 1980s, transplantation was becoming increasingly successful because of the development of immunosuppressive drugs and refined surgical techniques. As a result, more transplant centers proliferated throughout the country, and the number of patients who were candidates for transplantation rapidly expanded. Despite the UAGA of 1968, hospitals and transplant surgeons could not obtain enough organs for transplantation. Already, patients and their families were using media appeals to the public and to legislators in an effort to find donor organs. Professionals in the field realized that the demand could never be met without a centralized network to ensure that scarce donated organs were found and utilized to the greatest extent possible.

In reality, there were still few concrete laws focusing on the legal aspects of organ donation and transplantation. Already the public was expressing a concern that transplantation would be made available more readily to the wealthy. Furthermore, some suspected that wealthy foreigners were coming to the United States and essentially buying transplants, thus using up a scarce donated commodity that could save U.S. citizens' lives. In 1984 the U.S. Congress passed the National Organ Transplant Act (NOTA), which would prove to be among the most significant legislative plans to address a variety of issues in transplantation.

First and foremost, NOTA called for the establishment of a twenty-five-member multidisciplinary Task Force on Organ Transplantation and assigned it the goal of studying medical, legal, ethical, social, and economic issues pertaining to organ donation and transplantation. This task force ultimately concluded that the donor organ problem was partially a result of a lack of uniform standards in the field addressing such issues as quality assurance, organ procurement, and accountability. As a result, NOTA made recommendations for uniform standards for organ procurement, including establishment of the Uniform Determination of Death Act (UDODA) in all states. To help potentially increase the supply of donor organs, the task force also recommended the development of legislation that made requests for organs mandatory through various laws, such as making Medicare reimbursement contingent on a requirement to offer organ donation as an option in appropriate cases.

The UAGA also required that the Department of Health and Human Services create a specific unit to implement the act's various provisions, which resulted in the department's Division of Organ Transplant (now known as the Division of Transplantation). NOTA eventually led to the establishment of two vital organizations: the Organ Procurement and Transplantation Network and the Scientific Registry of Transplant Recipients. The latter registry was established to collect, store, analyze, and report on transplant data that would further transplant research.

NOTA also took one of the first steps to address a potential land mine in the field of transplantation. Specifically, it banned the sale of organs in any form for transplantation. The penalty for noncompliance included a fine of up to $50,000 and/or a prison sentence of up to five years.

The Organ Procurement and Transplantation Network

Next on the transplantation field's agenda was establishing a coordinated effort to procure and allocate organs. Following NOTA's lead, the

Organ Procurement and Transplantation Network (OPTN) was established as a united transplant network joining together all the various members of the transplant community. It is operated by a private, nonprofit
organization under federal contract, won by the United Network for
Organ Sharing (UNOS) in 1986. Under the guidelines established by the
OPTN, the primary goals of UNOS are twofold. First, UNOS is to
enhance the effectiveness of organ sharing and the equity in the national
system of organ allocation. Second, it focuses on increasing the supply of
donated organs available for transplantation. UNOS is also ultimately
responsible for matching donated organs with prospective recipients listed
on the UNOS organ transplant waiting list.

The OPTN also established membership criteria for various Organ Procurement Organizations (OPOs) throughout the country. For example, one
of the criteria is that OPOs must help in systematic efforts to obtain all use-
able organs from potential donors. The OPOs provide a crucial cornerstone
for the foundation supporting the entire transplant system. For example,
OPO organizations are largely responsible for approaching the families of
potential organ donors, putting them on the front line of the organ procurement system. Overall, approximately sixty OPOs exist throughout the
United States, with most focusing on an individual state, such as the Alabama Organ Center. However, some OPOs' jurisdictions cross state boundaries, such as the New York Organ Donor Network, which also includes
part of Pennsylvania. Once an OPO acquires an organ, it is placed within
the UNOS system for allocation. In addition to OPOs, all transplant centers
and tissue-typing laboratories belong to UNOS.

The Omnibus Budget Reconciliation Act of 1986

In the same year that UNOS was established, the federal government
passed the Omnibus Reconciliation Act (OBRA) of 1986. Although the
act primarily addressed nontransplant issues, such as the establishment of
the National Adoption Information Clearinghouse, it also included provisions addressing transplantation. In some ways, these provisions gave life
to the recommendations made by the Organ Transplantation Task Force.
For example, OBRA legally requires that all hospitals participating in
Medicare and Medicaid programs refer all potential organ donors to their
local OPO. It further mandates that all families of potential organ donors
become aware of their option to donate and that all transplant centers and
all OPOs be members of the Organ Procurement Transplant Network.
Still another provision established Medicare reimbursement for the cost of
immunosuppressive drugs for the first year following transplantation.

Uniform Anatomical Gift Act (UAGA) of 1987

In 1987 the National Conference of Commissioners on the Uniform State Laws drafted a new version of the 1968 UAGA to address the growing demands on the transplantation system. Specifically, the act sought to address the increasingly apparent inadequacies in organ procurement, especially in terms of encouraging voluntary donation of organs, as reported on by the Hastings Center. In addition to identifying inefficiencies in obtaining referrals of donors and in placing donating organs, the Hastings Center identified several key failures in organ procurement (Hastings Center, 1985):

1. The failure of people to sign written directives allowing their organs to be transplanted
2. The failure of police and emergency personnel to locate written directives at the site of accidents
3. The failure of medical personnel to recover organs on the basis of written directives
4. The failure to foster a system in which family members are systematically approached to inquire about organ donation
5. The failure to obtain adequate informed consent from family members.

To address these issues, the new UAGA differed from the 1968 version in several ways. In terms of increasing the likelihood of organ donation, perhaps the most important difference was that the new UAGA included a provision that sanctioned "presumed consent" in harvesting the recently deceased's organs. According to the new UAGA, if the prospective donor had made no objections, or if no objections by family members were known after a reasonable search had been conducted for next of kin, the hospital could assume presumed consent. However, only fourteen states adopted a provision allowing medical personnel to remove organs via the donor's presumed, rather than expressed, consent.

The new UAGA also addressed other failures noted by the Hastings Center report. It became mandatory that hospitals make routine inquiries and requests of patients concerning their wishes about organ donations. They also were required to ascertain whether an individual had previously signed an organ donor card. The UAGA instructed all emergency personnel, from paramedics to the police, to search accident victims for organ donor cards. Although failure to do so would not result in criminal charges, the act noted that those who failed to conduct such a search should be subject to administrative sanctions.

Further Government Efforts

Despite the several groundbreaking legislative efforts to increase the supply of donor organs, the need for organs continued to increase. A 1993 Gallup poll indicated that in America 85 percent of the people surveyed supported the idea of organ donation, with approximately 70 percent indicating that they were likely to donate their organs for transplantation. But these statistics belied the actual rate of organ donation because more than 50 percent of the time, family members refused to allow their loved ones' organs to be harvested for transplantation when their family members had not signed an organ donor card. In addition, many families were still not being approached about donation. The problem was profound, as revealed by the fact that a 250 percent increase occurred in the number of patients placed on the national organ transplant waiting list between 1996 and 1997, but only a 1 percent increase occurred in donation rates. This increase remained minimal despite the fact that in 1994 the National Coalition on Donation had been formed and had partnered with the Advertising Council to establish an ongoing national public education campaign to increase organ donation.

Realizing that further action was required, the Health Care Finance Administration (HCFA) under the Department of Health and Human Services took another look at the idea of linking federal funding for Medicare and Medicaid with the effort to increase organ donation. In 1998 the HCFA issued a rule, known as the "Hospital Conditions of Participation (CoP) for Organ Donation," requiring all hospitals that participate in Medicare to report in a timely manner all hospital deaths and imminent deaths to their local OPOs. HFCA also established several other transplant-related criteria that hospitals must comply with in order to receive financial reimbursement from Medicaid and Medicare, including the following:

- Establishing an agreement with an OPO
- Establishing an agreement with one tissue bank and at least one eye bank
- Working collaboratively with OPOs to ensure every family is offered the option of donation by OPO personnel or OPO-trained "designated requestors"
- Working with OPOs to educate hospital staff regarding the new conditions
- Collaborating with the OPOs in death-record reviews to improve identification of potential donors

In addition to federal interventions for organ procurement and allocation, many states were initiating their own laws addressing these issues. By 1988, forty-four states had already passed their own "required request" legislation.

National Donate Life Month

Numerous efforts have been made to increase the public's awareness of organ donation. In 1983, the U.S. Congress "authorized and requested" then President Ronal Reagan to establish a proclamation declaring April 22–29 each year as National Organ Donation Awareness Week. The third full week of April has since been the traditional time of observance for what soon became known as the National Organ and Tissue Donation Awareness Week. In 2003 President George W. Bush announced that the entire month of April would be observed as National Donate Life Month to further enhance efforts to raise public awareness of the critical need for organ, tissue, marrow, and blood donation. This change underscores the importance of donation and gives various transplant organizations throughout the country more time to sponsor public-awareness activities in their communities.

The Organ Donation Request Act of Illinois, for example, required hospitals in most circumstances to request organ-donation consent from next of kin and identified those relatives who could be contacted. In addition, the HCFA's CoP was based largely on Pennsylvania Act 102, which had already established a "routine referral" process in 1995.

Despite the CoP rule, compliance with OPTN policies was largely considered a voluntary decision. However, in 1999 the Department of Health and Human Services issued a formal regulation governing the network through its "Final Rule" for Organ Procurement and Transplantation. Effective March 16, 2000, the Final Rule had numerous provisions for organ procurement and allocation with the intent of encouraging organ donation, developing an allocation system that works on a nationwide basis, providing the basis for effective oversight of the OPTN by the federal government, and enhancing the information about transplantation given to patients, families, and health care workers.

The need for donor organs has also led to several congressional organ-donation bills in the early twenty-first century. The Organ Donation Improvement Act of 2001 authorizes federal grants or contracts to states, transplant centers, qualified OPOs, and other public and private entities for payment of travel and other expenses incurred by living donors or their family members. The Gift of Life Congressional Medal Act of 2001 established the designing and striking of a bronze medal to commemorate organ donors and their families and to foster donation.

On April 5, 2004, President George W. Bush signed into law the Organ Donation and Recovery Improvement Act (ODRIA) of 2004. This act focuses solely on improving organ donation rates and includes provisions to make live donation easier and more financially appealing. Overall, the act authorized a $25 million program focusing on such issues as educating the public about organ donation. The act's key initiatives include reimbursements for living donors for expenses related to organ donation, funds to establish public-awareness campaigns and for studies and demonstrations concerning organ donation, and authorization of potential grants to coordinate organ-donation activities of hospitals and OPOs.

AN ONGOING BATTLE

Efforts to improve organ donation rates finally began to show results in the twenty-first century. Typically, organ donation rates have increased approximately 1 to 2 percent per year. In 2003 organ donation was up by 4.3 percent, and 2004 saw an increase of 10.8 percent over the previous year. Furthermore, the first half of 2005 saw a 9.5 percent increase in organ donation over that same time period in 2004. In part, these increases were the result of an effort supported by the Department of Health and Human Services called the Organ Donation Breakthrough Collaborative, which focuses on improved efforts within participating transplant programs, donor hospitals, and organ-procurement organizations. One of the collaborative's aims is to foster the better utilization of each donor's organs by increasing the mean number of recipients transplanted per donor from 3.06 (2004 U.S. mean) to 3.75 or higher.

Nevertheless, despite federal and state initiatives and the increased efforts of OPOs and other organizations to improve organ donation rates, organ donation remains the most pernicious problem facing transplantation today. The number of people on the UNOS waiting list continues to skyrocket, far outpacing increases in donations. In 2005 organ donations supplied enough organs for only about 5 percent of those who needed them. In an editorial in the *Mayo Clinic Proceedings*, Susan Galandiuk and Sylvester Sterioff noted, "The vast majority of American hospitals have extremely low rates of organ donation, a problem compounded by not having advocates on their staff" (Galandiuk and Sterioff, 2005, p. 320).

One approach to solving the organ-donation problems encompasses a growing effort to foster live donor transplants for kidneys and livers. Nevertheless, this approach affects only a subset of patients and probably could never fulfill the full need even for these recipients. Furthermore, it raises ethical questions concerning potential harm to the healthy donor, which is discussed in a later chapter. Likewise, artificial organ technology, such as artificial hearts, has shown some promise. Still, this technology is in the developmental stage for the most part and serves primarily as a "bridge to transplantation," that is, keeping patients alive until an organ is available.

Another approach to solving the organ-donation problem is an increased effort to use more of the donor's organs and to widen the acceptable donor pool. This approach has led to "extended criteria" for organ and tissue donations, including increasing the age limit of donors in some cases and accepting donor organs obtained after cardiac death. The latter is referred to as non-heart-beating organ transplantation and uses donor organs from individuals whose deaths are the result of heart and respiratory-function failure rather than loss of whole brain function.

One of the long-term solutions to acquiring enough donor organs is to raise the awareness of the public concerning organ donation and thus convince people to sign organ donor cards, such as driver's license designations. According to Alden M. Doyle, Robert I. Lechler, and Laurence A. Turka in the *Journal of the American Society of Nephrology,*

> Much of this effort has centered on increasing the efficiency of the consent process through a variety of methods, including legislation to reaffirm donor gift laws, strengthening the organizational structure for the individual Organ Procurement Organizations (OPOs), and improving the way that the members of the hospital and OPO staff interface with the families of potential donors. (Doyle et al., 2004)

Several studies have also been conducted to differentiate between families who agree to organ donations and those who do not, and this has led to improved approaches to asking families for consent.

The transplantation of organs from animals, or xenotransplantation, such as pigs to humans, is an area of scientific research that some transplant professionals, including transplant pioneer Thomas E. Starzl, believe may one day eliminate the problem of not having enough organs to go around. However, scientists still must overcome many obstacles concerning issues of immunosuppression and organ rejection (see Chapter 4). Another avenue of investigations is to grow organs from dedifferentiated stem cells as an answer to the organ-shortage problems. Stem cells are cells that can replicate indefinitely and differentiate into other cells; stem cells also serve as a continuous source of new cells. These self-regenerating cells are found in bone marrow, testes, embryos, and umbilical cords.

Perhaps the most controversial suggestions involve abandoning the altruistic system of organ donation for a market-based approach in which organs are purchased like a commodity. Those in favor of this approach

---

A Look at the Numbers

The Organ Procurement and Transplantation Network keeps an ongoing tally of patients on the organ transplant waiting list, the number of transplants performed during the year, and the number of donor organs retrieved that year. Here's a look at the numbers from November 2005. Updated information can be found at http://www.optn.org/data/.

Organ donor waiting list candidates as of November 22, 2005*

Kidney	Pancreas	Kidney/Pancreas	Liver	
64,177	1,690	2,507	17,468	Total
Heart	Lung	Heart/Lung	Intestine	90,333
3,027	3,269	151	194	

*"All candidates" is less than the sum because of some patients waiting for multiple organs.

Transplants performed January–August 2005

Total	Deceased Donor	Living Donor
18,994	14,311	4,683

Donors recovered January–August 2005

Total	Deceased Donor	Living Donor
9,795	5,115	4,680

---

argue that it can be controlled to prevent favoritism toward the wealthy while increasing the likelihood that individuals and their families would agree to organ donation.

Despite the lack of donor organs, nearly 30,000 transplants were performed in 2004. Although these transplants have addressed the medical needs of many more people than what was once dreamed possible, they give rise to some questions as well: Who are the fortunate recipients of these valuable commodities? And how are they chosen?

CHAPTER 3

Organ Allocation: Establishing a Fair System

"I need a liver—Please help save my life," read several billboards on Houston highways in the summer of 2004. The billboards were part of a media campaign conducted by a 32-year-old Texas man and his wife to find a donor liver for the man, who was suffering from liver cancer. Although the United Network for Organ Sharing (UNOS) opposes advertising for organs, a spokesperson noted that such efforts do serve the purpose of raising awareness of the critical shortage of donor organs. The underlying message, of course, is that organ allocation would not be an issue if enough donor organs were available for all those in need.

As mentioned in the previous chapter, more than 90,000 people are on the organ transplant waiting list with approximately seventeen people dying each day because an organ is not available. On the surface, allocating organs would seem to be a straightforward process in which the transplant community would allocate organs to the sickest patients most in need of them. However, the "sickest-first" policy has drawbacks when dealing with a finite, rationed resource such as donor organs. For example, in the case just mentioned, the man did receive a donor organ when the family of a deceased donor directed that the organ go the Texas man. Nevertheless, the donor organ recipient died eight months after receiving the organ. His relatively quick demise illustrates one of the issues surrounding organ allocation—that is, whether or not the donated organ was put to best use. Some argued that the organ should have been allocated to someone else who could have benefited more in terms of long-term survival.

As transplantation became a viable and successful treatment for many diseases involving organ failure, the transplant community realized early on that numerous questions were bound to arise concerning allocation. As the field became successful and grew, the issue of who should receive a transplant came to the forefront. As expected, controversy has surrounded allocation policies from the very beginning and has only increased because of a progressively inadequate supply of donor organs. The current state of the debate is discussed in later chapters. This chapter focuses on exactly how organ allocation works in the United States and how allocation policies developed and evolved over the years.

LAYING THE FOUNDATION FOR ORGAN SHARING

Although the Uniform Anatomical Gift Act of 1968 laid the foundation for acquiring donor organs, it took another decade and a half before concrete national policies were set in place designed to ensure the equitable distribution of organs for transplantation. Prior to the passage of the National Organ Transplant Act of 1984, only a handful of transplant centers existed in the United States, and the sharing of donor organs was largely an informal, voluntary process. In fact, throughout the late 1950s and on through the 1960s, the early transplant pioneers acquired donor organs only from people who died in their hospital or immediate region. The sharing of organs on a national basis only occurred in the case of living-related donors.

Two primary factors made the long-distance sharing of cadaver donor organs a nonissue in the early days of transplantation. First of all, the field of transplantation was still considered in the experimental stages, and relatively few transplant operations were taking place. Second, the technology for preserving organs for any extended period of time did not yet exist. For example, organ preservation techniques today can safely preserve kidneys for up to forty-eight hours. However, in the early 1960s, such preservation was not possible. Surgeons had a small window of opportunity to successfully transplant an organ before it began to degrade because of ischemia, that is, localized tissue anemia resulting from obstruction or loss of the arterial blood inflow. Thus, the organ donor and the organ recipient had to be relatively close geographically.

By 1967, Folkert O. Belzer and colleagues had developed a solution called cryoprecipitated plasma (CPP) that could be pumped through an organ using a perfusion machine. In early experiments, Belzer found he could preserve dog kidneys for up to seventy-two hours and achieve 100 percent graft survival rates after autotransplantation, that is, transplanting the kidney back into the same animal. In August 1967, a patient suffering from amyloidosis (a disorder characterized by deposit of amyloid in organs or tissues; often secondary to chronic rheumatoid arthritis or tuberculosis) experienced renal failure and received a kidney seventeen hours after Belzer had placed it on his perfusion machine in the laboratory. The kidney functioned, although imperfectly. Nevertheless, hypothermic perfusion preservation of a human kidney was now a reality, meaning that kidneys could be transported over distances to patients almost anywhere in the United States.

Two years later, in 1969, David Hume at the Medical College of Virginia and Bernard Amos of Duke University developed the first organized kidney-sharing system with funding from the United States Public Health Service's Kidney Disease and Control Agency. Nine medical centers in a four-state area from Baltimore, Maryland, to Atlanta, Georgia, were recruited to participate in the organ-sharing system, which became known as the South-Eastern Regional Organ Procurement Program (SEROPP).

Although the system was partially made possible by the development of CPP, the impetus for it also came from tissue-typing advances in the 1960s that had led to better techniques for matching donor and recipient blood and tissues types. Both Hume and Amos had found that improved tissue typing increased graft survival for kidney recipients when good matches were obtained.

As with any resource, however, costs had to be taken into account. SEROPP quickly developed standard organ-acquisition charges to pay for the costs involved in recovering the organs and then sharing them between centers. Next, the organization established a fee for listing potential recipients on a waiting list. Over the ensuing years, SEROPP developed and expanded, was incorporated as a nonprofit organization in 1975, and was renamed the South-Eastern Organ Procurement Foundation (SEOPF) with eighteen charter members covering six states.

In addition to helping identify and define organ procurement costs, SEOPF made several other contributions that proved to be paramount in developing a nationwide organ procurement and allocation system. Among the most important of the program's contributions was the refinement of a computerized national waiting list and a sound methodology for matching donor kidneys with the proper recipients. Scientists within the program had developed cross-match recipient serum sample trays that allowed donors to be cross-matched through the computer program with potential recipients, no matter where the donors and recipients were located. This achievement greatly sped up the kidney-sharing process. Furthermore, SEOPF established educational programs as well as tissue typing and other manuals that it produced and distributed throughout the world.

In 1977 SEOPF was requested to coordinate the first long-distance donor-heart recovery for successful transplantation. This effort led the program to become the central collection center for data on solid organ transplants of all kinds. SEOPF collaborated with the American Kidney Fund in 1982 to become the clearinghouse for nationwide organ donation and referral efforts, with the goal of decreasing the wastage of organs. As a result of its pioneering efforts, SEOPF made it apparent that organ sharing had moved beyond the confines of geographical areas within the United States and that a similar program could be operated on a national scale.

CREATING A NATIONWIDE ALLOCATION SYSTEM

Although the successful efforts of SEOPF demonstrated that a national program of organ procurement and retrieval could be established, another factor played a prominent role in the creation of a government-approved and sponsored program. In a 1998 speech before the U.S. House of Representatives Human Resources Subcommittee, Claude Earl Fox, then the acting administrator of the Health Resources and Services Administration, recalled that ethical issues were a prime impetus in the move toward a national organ-allocation policy:

> Prior to passage of the National Organ Transplant Act, the distribution of organs was often unfair. Wealthy people or persons with special connections reportedly were able to manipulate the system so that they received organ transplants instead of people who were sicker and had been waiting far longer. Patients from foreign countries sometimes received lifesaving transplants while Americans died. After hearings and media reports had confirmed many of these allegations, Congress acted swiftly to establish a national system. (Fox, 1998)

Following the passage of the National Organ Transplant Act in 1984, the national Organ Procurement and Transplantation Network (OPTN) was established, and UNOS won the contract for both procuring and allocating organs in 1986 (see Chapter 2). A primary goal of UNOS has been to centralize a national organ-distribution system that assures that all patients have an equal chance to receive donor organs. As a part of that effort, a national U.S. Scientific Registry for Organ Transplantation was developed to compile and analyze data pertaining to all transplants performed in the United States. UNOS won the contract to administer this registry in 1987. As a national entity, UNOS's voluntary membership includes transplant centers, organ-procurement organizations (OPOs), independent tissue-typing laboratories, transplant consortia, professional and voluntary health organizations, and members of the general public.

The basic foundation for the operation of OPTN and subsequently UNOS came from the National Task Force on Organ Transplantation formed by the passage of the National Organ Transplant Act (NOTA). In its 1986 reports, *Organ Transplantation: Issues and Recommendations*, the task force made many recommendations based on its recognition that tradeoffs were going to be required, such as the tradeoff between medical urgency for an organ and the probability of its being successfully transplanted. As a result, it recommended a "thoughtful process of development of policies for allocation which takes into account both medical utility and good stewardship" (Task Force on Organ Transplantation, 1986, pp. 8–9). Furthermore, the task force suggested that the "selection of patients for transplant not be subject to favoritism, discrimination on the basis of race or sex, or ability to pay" (Task Force on Organ Transplantation, 1986, p. 44).

THE BASIC SYSTEM

The current UNOS Organ Center was first established in 1982 through SEOPF as the Kidney Center and became the Organ Center in 1984 as the result of more types of organs being transplanted successfully. The center's goal is to coordinate organ sharing among transplant centers, OPOs, and histocompatibility laboratories throughout the United States. This centralized computer network primarily operates to assist in gathering donor organ information, running a donor-recipient matching process, and then placing donor organs for transplantation. It also helps in the transportation of organs.

The matching of donor organs with recipients is a complex process that takes into consideration numerous factors, such as the medical compatibility between the donor and transplant candidate and how this may affect long-term survival. The transplant candidate's overall medical condition and its impact on the success of the transplant in terms of long-term survival is also an important factor. Overall, the matching and allocation system seeks to achieve the best possible survival rates and, in the process, make the most efficient use of its limited organ resources. The system is also designed to avoid taking into consideration such things as race, gender, religion, socioeconomic status, or personal and behavioral history into account when allocating organs.

Essentially, the matching process begins after a patient has been evaluated and deemed an appropriate candidate for transplantation. The patient's profile is then sent to a national patient waiting list "pool" of patients. When an organ is donated or becomes available, the OPO where the organ was donated sends information such as the organ's size, condition, and blood and tissue types to UNOS, which then generates a list of potential recipients, based on biological compatibility factors. The computer system then ranks candidates accordingly, also factoring in various clinical characteristics of the patients. Major factors taken into consideration in allocating the organ include age, blood type, medical urgency, the amount of time the patient has spent on the waiting list, and the distance between the donor and potential recipient. Then specialists in organ placement at the OPO or the UNOS Organ Center contact the transplant centers that have patients who are high on the local list.

According to the UNOS policy, the transplant center has one hour to make its decision regarding whether to accept the organ for its patients. Often, the center with the top patient does not accept the organ for various reasons. For example, the patient may not be healthy enough at the moment to undergo a transplant. Other medical-biological factors that may preclude transplantation include having high antibody levels that prove to be incompatible to the donor organ and would cause rejection. In addition, the patient must be available and willing to be transplanted immediately. If an organ is refused, UNOS continues to offer the organ to patients at other centers until it is accepted.

ORGAN TYPE AND WAITING TIMES

All organs and all organ transplants are not created equal. In fact, each organ has its own complex set of medical criteria for matching. For example, matches for the heart, liver, and lungs focus on blood type and body size whereas the matching process for pancreas and kidneys also consider genetic tissue. In almost all cases, the basic allocation policies described in the previous section apply, and normally organs are allocated locally first and then by a specific sequence of areas or zones. The following is a brief overview of important factors in the UNOS allocation process that can affect waiting times for each type of organ:

- Heart—Potential heart-transplant recipients also receive a status code based on medical urgency.
- Lungs—Lung-transplant candidates are grouped together for both single- and double-lung transplants and are given the same priority status. If a lung is given to a patient needing a single-lung transplant, the other lung is then allocated to another patient awaiting a single-lung transplant.
- Heart/Lung—Heart/lung candidates are placed on the individual patient waiting list for each organ. When a patient is eligible to receive a donor heart or lung, then the other organ (either the heart or the lung) is also allocated to the same candidate from the same donor.

- Liver—Those candidates waiting for a donor liver are given a status code or point system taken from the mortality risk score corresponding to their degree of medical urgency. This is based on scores derived from the Model for End-Stage Liver Disease/Pediatric End-Stage Liver Disease (MELD/PELD). Candidates are prioritized to receive livers according to the MELD/PELD scores. The code ranges from 1, which is the most urgent need, to 7, which is the least urgent. Livers are not offered to candidates who rank 7 in the system.
- Kidney—The characteristics of the kidney-transplant candidate and the kidney-donor are taken into consideration together in the allocation of kidneys. The policy is based primarily on histocompatibility. Also taken into consideration is whether the recipient is a child.
- Pancreas—Candidates are divided into those awaiting an isolated pancreas, those in need of a kidney–pancreas combination, or those waiting for a combined solid organ-islet transplant from the same donor. Because the pancreas remains viable for transplantation for a limited amount of time outside of the donor's body compared with organs such as the liver, the allocation policy includes a facilitated allocation sequence that comes into effect five hours after the donor organ is first offered. This process includes offering the pancreas to patients who previously had not received an offer. Because these organs are less desirable overall, only a few transplant centers participate in the facilitated program.
- Intestinal—Candidates for transplant of stomach, small intestine, large intestine or for transplant of any portion of the gastrointestinal tract receive a status code according to their medical condition. Size-compatibility also plays a large role in the allocation process.

FINE-TUNING THE SYSTEM

Despite the basic foundation for organ procurement and allocation first established by SEOPF and efforts to maintain an ethical approach to the fair sharing of organs as stated by the Task Force on Organ Transplantation and initiated by OPTN and UNOS, the allocation of organs in the United States has remained one of the most contentious aspects of transplantation. In a 2003 position statement on organ allocation, the American Society of Transplantation (AST) noted that it supported the UNOS system but added that continued evaluation was necessary in order to make sure it operated optimally and efficiently. This belief has generally been agreed upon by all involved in organ transplantation, from the medical community to the government. As a result, organ allocation has remained

---

Living Donor Allocation

One alternative that has helped with the shortage of cadaveric organs (organs that come from deceased donors) is living donor transplants. Kidneys represent the most frequent type of living-donor organ donation. However, refined surgical techniques and improved postdonation medical care has made it possible for people to donate a segment of their liver, which will regenerate. Other types of living donor transplants are much more rare and include donation of a lobe of one lung and donation of a portion of the intestine or pancreas. In very rare cases, an individual who receives a heart/lung transplant from a deceased donor may have his or her healthy heart given to an individual waiting for a heart transplant and, as a result, is considered a living donor.

Most living donor transplants are directed donations in which the donors are relatives or friends of the transplant recipients or somehow closely associated with the recipient through church or some other community organization. Much more rare is the nondirected living donations, sometimes referred to as anonymous, altruistic, or stranger-to-stranger living donation. These organs are allocated under direction of the United Network for Organ Sharing organ allocation policies.

Although living organ donors can direct their organs to be used for a certain individual, they cannot sell their organs. Furthermore, there is a growing debate over people soliciting for live donations through advertising or other means. Most organizations, including UNOS and the American Society of Transplant Surgeons, oppose this practice as subverting the fair policies of organ allocation.

---

under close scrutiny from the very beginning, and the rules regarding allocation have been revised as part of an ongoing effort to improve the process and make it as fair as possible.

As early as 1988, only two years after UNOS was established and a set of medical criteria was in place to direct organ allocation, questions concerning the equity of organ allocation were raised. As a result, Congress amended the 1984 National Organ Transplant Act legislation to clarify the process through the Organ Transplant Act Amendments of 1988. The amended legislation stated that both transplant hospitals and OPOs must be members of OPTN and must abide by its policies. It also stressed that organs were to be allocated according to established medical criteria and that allocation systems should focus on allocation among patients and not on transplant centers themselves.

Another report by the House Committee on Energy and Commerce urged the Department of Health and Human Services (HSS) secretary to monitor the allocation process more closely. The primary reason for this recommendation stemmed from the early task force's final report. The report had emphasized the importance of a national system of organ allocation but had not mandated such a system. Instead, it noted that a national system could be created through various regional centers instead of one location. However, questions arose over whether or not a national system of equitable distribution was really a priority in the transplant community. As a result, Congress passed the Transplant Amendments Act of 1990, once again stressing that the OPTN was to assist in ensuring that organs would be distributed nationwide in an equitable fashion to transplant patients. The act also required the OPTN to submit transplant center–specific data to HHS as a part of an effort to monitor performance and efforts to meet allocation goals.

The urgency of the problem was illustrated the following year when the Office of the Inspector General of the U.S. Department of Health and Human Services issued a report titled *The Distribution of Organs for Transplantation: Expectations and Practices.* The transplantation waiting list in 1991 had more than 20,000 patients on it. Although this number is less than a quarter of the number of patients who were on the waiting list by 2005, there was already growing concern over the fairness of the organ-allocation process. The report acknowledged that some progress had been made in establishing a national system. Nevertheless, it pointed out that the program at that time was falling far short of expectations of creating a cooperative system based on the best interests of patients nationwide waiting for a transplant. The report focused primarily on the area of kidney transplantation, which continues to account for the most number of transplants performed. It noted several inequalities in organ allocations, such as much longer waiting times for transplants at some centers as opposed to others. Another inequality was that blacks were waiting almost twice as long for transplants as whites. The report further pointed out that in the various OPO service areas few transplant centers were collaborating to develop a common list of transplant candidates. There was also a lack of collaboration pertaining to a distribution of organs to candidates on a first-come, first-served basis nationwide within the medical criteria rules.

Overall, it appeared that the organ distribution was controlled primarily by the individual transplant centers and occurred primarily within the OPOs' individual service areas. In other words, the distribution of organs from donors to recipients remained highly localized. In the final analyses, the report pointed out that only about 22 percent of kidneys procured for transplantation were being shared nationally.

THE FINAL RULE ON ORGAN ALLOCATION

In 1997 John Neylan, then president-elect of the American Society of Transplant Physicians (ASTP), made a presentation at an Institute of Medicine meeting in which he outlined some of the problems that persisted with organ allocation:

> Organ allocation, without a doubt, has engendered the most contentious public policy debate regarding transplantation in years. Throughout this debate, it has been observed that the variation in criteria physicians use to list a patient for transplant has contributed to the inconsistencies in waiting times among patients across the country. Furthermore, there is concern that, because of long waiting times in certain regions, there is a pressure on transplant programs to list patients early, before they actually require transplantation, a practice referred to as "waiting list inflation." While many other factors contribute to these regional differences including OPO productivity and the available supply of local donors, the increasing discrepancy between the short supply of donor organs and expanding list of patients in need has spurred a growing demand to ensure that the organ allocation system is efficient and equitable. (Neylan, 1997)

Officials within the Health and Human Services agency were also growing increasingly concerned that organs were not being distributed in an equitable manner, especially across state lines. In 1998 then Department of Health and Human Services (DHHS) Secretary Donna Shalala ordered that major changes were to be made in the process of allocating donor organs. The three major changes proposed under the Final Rule on Organ Allocation were as follows:

1. Eliminate geography as a factor in determining who gets an organ.
2. Develop uniform national criteria for placing patients on transplant lists on the basis of measurable medical criteria.
3. Develop uniform national criteria based on measurable medical criteria for ranking those patients by need.

In addition to these changes, the new rule would give authority to the DHHS secretary to review and ultimately approve OPTN policies. Shalala also wanted to change the makeup of the OPTN Board of Directors and allow no more than half of its members to be transplant surgeons or transplant physicians in order to ensure that the policy-making process was not dominated by transplant professionals.

Patient and Public Input on UNOS Policies

According to the United Network for Organ Sharing (UNOS), transplantation may be the only medical field in the United States in which patients and the general public can take a formal role in helping to make policies. Both patients and the general public are encouraged to bring issues concerning organ allocation and other aspects of transplantation to the attention of the Organ Procurement Transplant Network and UNOS. Committees then consider whether a new policy or a policy change should be made. If a recommendation is made to create or change a policy, then both patients and the public are encouraged to comment on the proposal. These comments are also taken under consideration before the organizations' committees make a final recommendation concerning policy creation or change to the OPTN/UNOS Board of Directors. If the board votes to approve or change a new policy, then OPTN/UNOS submits the policy to the Department of Health and Human Services (HHS) for review and approval. Any organ allocation policy is voluntary within the various members of UNOS until the HHS approves it.

The issue of regional OPOs and geography has remained a highly debated topic for several reasons. The UNOS system of allocation is based on eleven geographic regions encompassing sixty-three local areas within them that are serviced by various OPOs. In addition, some geographic regions could have as many as twelve OPOs, such as region 3, which included the states of Alabama, Arkansas, Florida, Georgia, Louisiana, and Mississippi. It should be noted that the proposed Final Rule on Organ Allocation was largely directed toward issues concerning liver transplants. After 1991 the "most urgent" category had been eliminated from liver-allocation policy, and it appeared that sharing of livers outside the UNOS regions was being discouraged. As a result, under the UNOS system, a liver could be given to a less critically ill patient in a local OPO instead of a more critically ill patient who was outside of the same OPO but still within a geographic area in which the liver could be transported quickly enough to remain viable for a transplant. Shalala was insisting that the organ be treated as a national resource and be given to the most critically ill patient regardless of the patient's place of residence or place of listing as long as the organ could be transported to the patient in time.

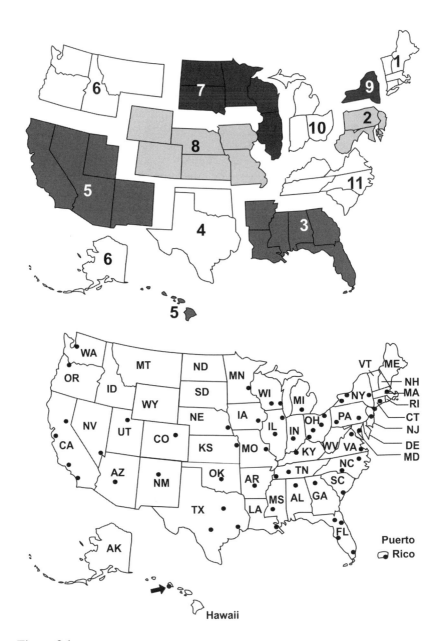

Figure 3.1
The national UNOS membership is divided into eleven geographic regions in the United States (top map). Organs are allocated first according to these regions and the various areas within them. There are approximately fifty-nine Organ Procurement Organizations, or OPOs, operating as part of the Organ Procurement and Transplantation Network (OPTN) in these various regions (bottom map).

UNOS opposed the Final Rule and the government's intervention on the basis that the proposed rule inappropriately placed government within the boundaries of the patient–physician relationship. UNOS also claimed that the disparity in waiting times for patients in certain geographical regions and areas was not as high as the government indicated, pointing out that the sickest patients on life support who were expected to live less than a week had an average waiting period, nationwide, of four to six days for a liver. Another objection against a policy that gave organs to the sickest patients on a nationwide basis argued that it would be counterproductive to the goal of saving and prolonging as many lives as possible. If the sickest people predominantly get the most organs, then most transplant patients would be very sick, resulting in more people ultimately dying because these patients are the least likely to survive a transplant.

The firestorm of controversy that resulted from the Final Rule proposal also included top congressional leaders, the courts, and state governors. Another concern among those opposed to the changes was the contention that more organs would be diverted to larger transplant centers, thus forcing smaller centers to close and making it more difficult for the sicker and poorer to reach a transplant center. Many also felt that such a turn of events could negatively affect organ donation in these areas. For example, former Wisconsin governor Tommy Thompson suspected that Wisconsin's highly effective organ-donation program would be hurt when local citizens understood that organs donated within the state could be transported to other states that had less successful donation programs. He eventually filed a suit against the DHHS claiming that the secretary had overstepped her authority. The suit was ultimately dismissed.

Despite UNOS's objection to the Final Rule, not all parties, including UNOS members, were against the changes. Primarily, the larger transplant centers and the states where they resided were in favor of the rule. For example, the University of Pittsburgh Medical Center and the Thomas E. Starzl Transplantation Institute located at the University of Pittsburgh favored the rule. The institute is perhaps the most well-established transplant center in the world and took in desperately sick patients who represented some of the most difficult cases in transplantation. As a result, the Starzl Institute had a much longer waiting list of sicker patients than most other centers and needed more organs to save these patients' lives.

The controversy surrounding the proposed Final Rule grew precipitously as opposing factions organized large coalitions. For example, the University of Pittsburgh organized a coalition in favor of the rule that was composed of the American Liver Foundation, the National Transplant Action Committee, the Minority Organ and Tissue Transplant Education Program, and the

Transplant Recipients International Organization. On the other hand, UNOS garnered support against the rule from the American Transplant Surgeons Society and the Patient Access to Transplantation Coalition.

Because of the controversy, Congress suspended the rule temporarily after many states complained. An amended version of the Final Rule, however, went into effect on March 16, 2000. As passed, the rule still specifically noted that allocation of organs should not be based on the potential transplant recipients' place of residence or listing and laid out guidelines for government and transplant professionals throughout the country. These guidelines required future organ allocation policies to be based on shared, or common, medical criteria and not on what some have referred to as "accidents of geography." Nevertheless, the ruling did not require a single nationwide list. And even though UNOS made some adjustments to its sharing procedures, true organ sharing on a national basis has yet to be achieved.

The debate over whether the Final Rule represents an intrusion by "Big Brother" did not go away completely once the rule was implemented. Nevertheless, the organ-allocation policy over recent years has largely followed the Final Rule's objective of making allocation policies more strongly based on objective and measurable medical criteria. As noted in a continuing education article by Gwen Mayes posted on the Medscape Web site,

> It is a process that is evolving gradually, but also one that is providing a strong and valid foundation upon which to establish policy. A 3-pronged approach has been key: (1) HRSA [Health Resources and Services Administration] provides the regulatory oversight; (2) the OPTN provides the formula and process for policy formation; and (3) the SRTR [Scientific Registry for Transplant Recipients] provides the statistical analysis and review of the policies to determine their compliance and fit with the federal mandate. (Mayes, 2005)

CONTINUING THE REVIEW

As long as a shortage of donor organs exists, allocation policies will continue to be questioned and reviewed to preserve the best aspects of the current system while correcting inequities and problems within it. For example, the kidney remains the most transplanted organ, with more than 60,000 of those on the transplant waiting list in 2005 needing kidneys. As a result, UNOS in 2005 began the process of reviewing the complex formula that has guided kidney allocation almost from the very beginning of successful kidney transplants. To make the best possible use of this limited resource, the review may result in new factors being applied to the kidney-allocation formula pertaining to both the donor and the recipient as suggested by the Kidney Allocation Review Subcommittee. One example of a possible change to the formula would be to consider that each individual kidney has a different biological life expectation that could better biologically suit one patient over another.

Policymakers and medical professionals have grappled with organ-allocation policies for more than thirty years. Throughout this time the fundamental question behind these policies has remained the same: who should benefit when someone makes the altruistic decision to donate organs upon death? In the end, the ultimate solution to the problem is to increase the availability of organs, either through human donors or via other sources, such as organs from animals, known as xenotransplantation. The next chapter discusses xenotransplantation and other advances in transplantation that are changing the field's future and raising new ethical questions.

CHAPTER 4

Advances and the Future of Transplantation

"Healing is not a science, but the intuitive art of wooing nature," noted W.H. Auden in his poem "The Art of Healing." If true, few areas in medical science over the past decade have wooed nature better than transplant practitioners. Transplantation is now the preferred and most effective treatment for patients with end-stage organ failure. Transplant recipients are living longer than ever and with a better quality of life. A field once practiced and researched by a handful of pioneering surgeons today encompasses a wide array of disciplines, such as immunologists, internists, geneticists, pathologists, biologists, and HLA (tissue-typing) experts. New areas of investigation include xenotransplantation, stem cell biology, cloning, artificial organs, and tissue engineering.

Stem cell transplants are another promising area of development and may offer new treatment approaches for a wide range of medical problems, from neurological disorders such as Parkinson's disease to repairing damaged hearts. Efforts are ongoing to transplant entire body parts, and between 2000 and 2005 surgeons around the world performed more than twenty-five hand transplants. Transplantation also made headline news worldwide in 2005 when a team of surgeons in France performed the first partial face transplant on a disfigured woman.

Despite promising results in many areas and the potential to offer even a wider range of patients new hope, many of these efforts are controversial and have engendered debate. This chapter focuses on some of the most important advances and research efforts in transplantation and how they may affect the future of a discipline that is still in its relative infancy.

IMMUNE SUPPRESSION AND TOLERANCE

Talk to almost anyone in the field of transplantation, and they will point to inducing long-term tolerance to transplanted organs as the field's "holy grail." Although phenomenal advances have been made in developing immunosuppressive drugs to reduce organ rejection, these powerful antirejection drugs come with many problems of their own. For example, the use of steroids such as prednisone can cause side effects ranging from weight gain to serious complications such as diabetes, osteoporosis, and muscle atrophy. Perhaps the most serious complication is increased susceptibility to bacterial and viral infections, which is more life threatening in this population than usual because of reduced immune-system functioning.

One of the most successful and widespread immunosuppressive drugs has been cyclosporine, which includes such common side effects as headaches, blurred vision, high blood pressure, and decreased kidney function. Tacrolimus, also known as FK506 or Prograf, is used to prevent rejection of organs and to treat acute (rapid) or chronic (long-term) rejection episodes. In addition to having side effects similar to those of cyclosporine, tacrolimus can elevate blood sugar levels. Immunosuppressive drugs also have other significant side effects, including mouth sores, gastrointestinal problems such as stomach upset and diarrhea, increased blood cholesterol levels, and decreased white blood cell counts. People taking these drugs appear to have a higher risk of developing tumors and cancer. Another concern is these drugs' potential long-term effects, which are currently unknown given that relatively few people have taken them over an extended period.

In an effort to more effectively and safely suppress the immune systems, transplantation professionals are working with immunosuppressive drugs in a number of ways. For example, studies are underway in lung transplantation using cyclosporine in an aerosol spray along with other immunosuppressive drugs in pill form. Early results have shown that delivery of the drug directly to the transplanted lungs through the use of an inhaler may help cut the rates of both early and long-term rejection. Another approach has been to wean transplant recipients off of certain drugs used in the immunosuppressive regimen. One weaning approach seeks to avoid giving patients high doses of multiple drugs over an extended period of time. Rather, the patient receives a one-time dose of a drug that depletes important immune system cells just hours before transplantation. After the operation is completed, lower-than-usual doses of just one antirejection drug are given beginning the day after transplantation. If no rejection occurs within ninety days, then the weaning process begins.

Scientists are also working in the areas of tolerance induction and chimerism. Tolerance induction is an attempt to achieve a peaceful coexistence between the recipient's immune system and the foreign donor graft in an effort to enhance long-term graft and patient survival, decrease the need for retransplantation, and perhaps greatly reduce or eliminate the need for immunosuppressants. Scientists have discovered that transplant recipients who have lived from ten to thirty years with a transplanted organ develop an intermingling of white blood cells from both the recipient and donor immune system. This coexistence of donor and recipient cells is called "chimerism," named after the Greek mythological beast called the Chimera, which had a lion's head, a goat's body, and a serpent's tail. Studies in this area, which include the infusion of donor marrow during organ transplantation to significantly boost "natural" chimerism, may be a crucial step in the development of whole organ tolerance without the need for immunosuppressive drugs. Not only would this approach benefit patients by reducing serious drug side effects, but it possibly could reduce the need for retransplantation as well, thus increasing the organ supply.

XENOTRANSPLANTATION

Because of the shortage of donor organs, xenotransplantation—the transplantation of organs between different species—represents a major pioneering effort in transplantation research. If successful in developing xenotransplantation, such as the use of pig organs for transplantation into humans, scientists could virtually eliminate numerous transplantation patient deaths resulting from a donor organ not arriving in time. Considering the dearth of donor organs, many scientists consider xenotransplantation to be critical to the field's future.

The first xenotransplantation experiments date back to the 1960s, when Dr. Thomas E. Starzl performed a series of baboon-to-human kidney transplants with little success. He reinitiated the studies in the early 1990s with two baboon-to-human liver transplants, but one patient died a little more than two months later, and another survived only about four weeks because of infections and kidney failure. Although the patients did not die from organ rejection, Dr. Starzl and most of his colleagues agreed that much more had to be learned about xenotransplantation before proceeding.

Today, xenotransplantation research efforts are focusing largely on pig organs, which are remarkably similar to human organs. Pigs also are thought to be better donors than baboons and other primates. Primates such as baboons, for example, are close species relatives to humans and harbor many viruses that may be easily transmitted to people. Pigs are also considered to be generally "healthier" than primates. They can be bred easily and produce many offspring during one birthing period, meaning that far more organs would be available for harvesting. In addition, people generally have fewer moral objections to using pigs than they have to using primates given that pigs are already slaughtered for food.

Initial studies with pig donor organs in the 1980s led to prompt rejection of the organs, which researchers later discovered was due to a sugar called galactose found on the surface of pig blood vessels and quickly targeted for destruction by immune system antibodies. To overcome this obstacle, scientists turned to the idea of genetically altering pigs. In 2002, PPL Therapeutics, Inc., created the world's first cloned pigs lacking the gene for the galactose sugar that was associated with hyperacute, or immediate, rejection. Genetic researchers are attempting to develop new generations of genetically altered pigs in which additional modification of genes will protect even further against rejection by the human immune system.

In addition to whole organs, pig islet cells (see page 60) are under research to treat diabetes and pig brain cells to treat neurological diseases. Scientists also point out that the initial use of these organs might not be as a permanent organ replacement but rather as a temporary replacement, or "bridge," until a suitable human donor organ can be found.

In addition to organ rejection, there are other concerns about using pigs as organ donors and cell transplant donors. Similar to the use of primates, some people are concerned about the possibility of a viral infection passing from pigs into humans. Other ethical concerns include the overall safety of genetically modifying animal organs for placement in humans and the best allocation of health resources.

Nevertheless, scientists point out that xenotransplantation has many potential advantages over using cadaveric human donor organs. Animals and their organs can be developed transgenically, that is, with genetically modified genes. For example, research is underway to insert human genes into pig organs in order to produce proteins that the transplant recipient's immune system will recognize as "human." Animals such as pigs could also be scheduled for death and organ donation exactly at the time the donor organ is needed. In addition, some animals are not susceptible to some human diseases, such as the case of baboons, whose livers are resistant to hepatitis B.

ARTIFICIAL ORGANS

Scientists have long been working on another approach to help resolve the organ shortage problem. Scientists first began developing artificial kidneys in the 1920s in the form of dialysis machines used outside of the patient's body. Today, more than 300,000 people in the United States with end-stage renal disease receive dialysis daily. For many years, artificial organs were large machines, such as the first clinically successful heart-lung pump in 1953, which were connected to patients either intermittently or on a continuous basis.

Totally implantable devices, however, were beyond the realm of that era's technology. In 1982, Seattle dentist Barney Clark was the first person to be implanted with an artificial heart. He received a Jarvik-7 and survived 112 days. Over the subsequent decades, artificial heart development has continued. Despite progress, devising a technologically complex, totally implantable, and completely reliable device to replace the function of the human heart has proved difficult. Research has largely focused on using artificial devices as a bridge to transplantation.

One of the most successful types of artificial heart is the left ventricular assist (LVAD) device, which helps maintain the heart's pumping ability by "assisting" the heart's left ventricle, which is the large heart chamber that pumps blood through the body. These temporary implantable pumps can keep patients alive for longer periods as they await a heart transplant. Outcomes have been good, and the majority of patients receiving these devices are surviving and doing well. As a result, researchers are looking into these devices as permanent implants to replace transplantation in some heart patients.

Total heart replacement devices for people suffering from biventricular heart failure are also under development but have yet to achieve good long-term results. Because of the highly experimental nature of these devices, patients who become candidates to receive them are usually ineligible for heart transplantation, not able to be helped by any other therapy, and have a high probability of dying within a relatively short time span.

Despite limited success with totally implanted devices, artificial organ research continues with devices such as the implantable membrane oxygenator, a type of "artificial lung" that helps oxygenate the blood of people suffering from acute respiratory distress syndrome. For the most part, most observers agree that artificial organ development is potentially beneficial for many patients. As with most aspects of medical care in the twenty-first century, issues of fair allocation and cost continue to be problematic. Some feel that putting a large medical effort into developing such machines may be placing too great an emphasis on "rescuing" patients who are among the most severely ill, thus reducing the emphasis on the utility of achieving the best medical outcomes for the most number of people in a fair manner.

ISLET CELL TRANSPLANTATION

Cellular transplantation, which involves transplanting the cellular components of organs instead of entire organs, is another promising area of development in transplantation. Perhaps the most advanced area of cellular transplantation is islet cell transplantation, which represents one of the most promising treatments for people with Type 1 diabetes, especially those who have problems controlling their blood sugar levels with daily insulin injections.

Islet cells are the insulin-producing beta cells found in a nest of pancreatic cells called the Islets of Langerhans. Experiments to treat diabetes with islet cells began in the 1960s, and by the early 1970s, scientists were getting positive results in animal models. In these experiments, scientists found that the transplanted islet cells continued to monitor sugar levels and regulate insulin to normalize blood glucose levels as the body's needs changed—after eating, for example. However, making the therapy work in humans proved frustrating and slow as over the next three decades researchers struggled with low success rates. The problem was that most transplanted islet cells taken from a donor pancreas failed within a few months when transplanted into humans.

Antirejection drugs that were used to allow the transplant recipient to accept the donor cells were part of the problem. Unfortunately, in humans these cells interfere with the insulin's effectiveness. However, in 1999 researchers at the University of Alberta in Edmonton, Canada, made a major advance. They developed the Edmonton Protocol by using special enzymes to remove islets from the donor pancreas and another method to prepare the extremely fragile cells. With the addition of improved immunosuppressive drugs, the researchers found that they were achieving a 100 percent success rate in clinical trials as opposed to the previous 8 percent success rate. The approach is now being studied around the world.

Islet cell transplantation promises many advantages for controlling diabetes. For example, the procedure itself does not require the extensive operation necessary for organ transplants. Rather than spending hours in the operating room undergoing a major operation, the patient undergoes a relatively minor procedure that involves the administration of a local anesthetic, after which a thin needle is inserted into the main blood vessel in the liver, called the portal vein. The islet cells are injected into the vein. If the cells develop a blood supply (by attaching to new blood vessels) and begin producing insulin, the patient may no longer have to undergo frequent blood glucose measurements or take daily insulin injections. It can also more fully protect against serious long-term complications associated with diabetes, such as heart disease, stroke, kidney disease, and nerve and eye damage.

Despite the ease of the procedure, however, islet cell recipients must take immunosuppressants and deal with their potentially adverse side effects. Islet cell transplantation also shares another disadvantage with organ transplants in that the cells are retrieved from donor organs, which are in limited supply. A typical procedure requires about one million islets, which is the equivalent of two donor organs. Scientists are investigating several approaches to overcoming this obstacle. One approach is to treat pancreatic islet cells with hepatocyte growth factor (HGF), which they hope will dramatically reduce the number of these cells needed for transplants to reverse Type 1 diabetes. Other options under investigation include the use of islet cells from pigs and growing insulin-producing cells in the laboratory from stem cells.

BIOARTIFICIAL ORGANS AND CELL ENGINEERING

Efforts in cell engineering and bioartificial organs seek to mimic the biological world and have been applied to organs such as the liver and pancreas, as well as to parts of the nervous system, skin, blood vessels, cartilage, bone, and muscle. Skin substitutes that incorporate living cells cultured on a biodegradable fabric have been most successful.

Still in the early stages of development, bioartificial organs currently involve the design, modification, growth, and maintenance of living cells or tissues encapsulated in natural or synthetic scaffolds. For example, pancreatic islet-cell transplantation for diabetes patients includes research efforts in this area. The membrane and scaffolding can provide viral protection and block host antigens, which the immune system uses to detect and attack foreign invaders. In the case of pancreatic islet-cell transplantation, the cells can also be genetically modified to include suicide genes for the destruction of cells or their secretions in case of malfunction or transplant failure.

Nanotechnology, an engineering field that focuses on working with particles on the nanometer scale of 0.1 to 100 nm, also holds promise for bioartificial engineering of organs and other body structures. A nanometer is about one millionth of a millimeter, and some scientists believe that it may be useful for sensing and controlling implants and for inducing, maintaining, and replacing missing function that cannot be readily substituted with a living cell.

One approach in bioartificial organ engineering is to mold an encapsulating structure out of biodegradable materials, insert human cells (perhaps the patient's own stem cells), inject them in an area such as the liver or kidney, and wait for the artificial scaffolding to degrade and leave behind functioning organ cells. In essence, some believe that patients can grow their own organs by donating cells from their own body to be grown in the laboratory and then reinserted in the donor's body. Another example of bioartificial engineering is the artificial "bionic" liver, a bridge-to-transplantation research effort that uses a tiny pump with a chamber containing human liver cells. Connected to the patient with a catheter, the liver cells organize themselves into a type of "mini-liver" to clean the patient's blood like the natural organ. Using a process called organogenesis—a natural process in which the ectoderm, endoderm, and mesoderm develop into internal organs—scientists are also researching how to "grow" lungs for transplantation.

Even though they are in their relative infancy, cell engineering and bioartificial organs are under close scrutiny. Because these cells can be engineered with animal cells and genes, some raise concerns about long-term medical and species impact. Although the goal is not to create chimeric people like the half-human and half-beast characters in the H.G. Wells science fiction novel *The Island of Dr. Moreau*, questions remain about the long-term psychological impact and resultant quality of life.

The introduction of nanotechnology raises questions of placing submicroscopic "machines" in the human body. For example, carbon nanotubes and fullerenes (buckyballs) are nanoparticles of carbon that are strong candidates for nanotechnology use. However, a Southern Methodist University researcher found that exposing fish to fullerenes for forty-eight hours at a moderate dose might cause extensive brain damage. Furthermore, scientists found that the fish had altered liver-gene markers, raising questions about changing human physiology at a fundamental level.

STEM CELL TRANSPLANTATION

Although the words "magic" and "science" are seldom used together, stem cells may be as close to "magical" as any biological component of the human body. These immature, uniform cells have the ability to morph, or differentiate, into any kind of cell and tissue. Thus, in the realm of cellular transplantation, transplanted stem cells might effectively replace damaged or diseased tissue almost anywhere in the body, from the brain to the heart and liver. As a result, stem cells have the potential to be a renewable source of therapeutic cells used to treat a variety of conditions, including Parkinson's disease, Alzheimer's disease, and spinal cord injuries. For example, in the case of Parkinson's disease, surgeons have injected stem cells into the area of the brain that produces dopamine, which is not produced effectively

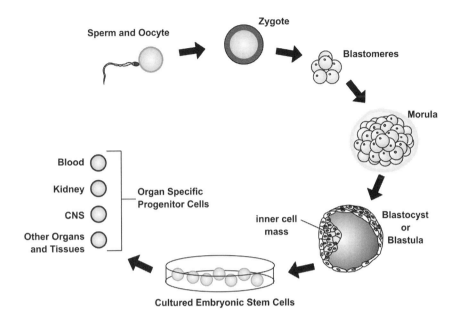

Figure 4.1

Embryonic stem cells: A zygote, or single cell, is formed at the time of conception and subsequently grows into a cluster of totipotent blastomeres, which result
from the cleavage of fertilized eggs. Cell division continues, first producing the
morula, a solid mass of twelve or more blastomeres that enter the uterus when in
their natural female human environment. The next stage of development is the
blastocyst, or blastula, a hollow ball within which the placenta, supporting tissues, and inner cell mass are formed. Embryonic stem cells can be produced from
placing inner cell masses on a plastic dish and culturing them in incubation
ovens. With further culturing, these pluripotent embryonic stem cells can form
into various types of human tissue.

in a Parkinson's patient. Arthritis, diabetes, heart disease, and other maladies
are also being targeted for treatment.

The medical field has practiced stem cell transplantation for more than
thirty years in the form of bone marrow transplants, which contain blood-
forming stem cells. In addition to red blood cells, stem cells can form white
blood cells, which are important components of the immune system and
help fight infections. For example, bone marrow and peripheral stem cells
(that is, stem cells in the circulating blood similar to those found in bone
marrow) have been used to treat some cancers, including leukemia and
lymphoma, as well as conditions such as anemia and inherited immune disorders. Bone marrow transplants are also being studied in organ transplantation

to induce tolerance to transplanted organs by creating bone marrow chimerism, which is a mixture of white blood cells from both the donor and the recipient that results in the immune system not recognizing the transplanted organ as "foreign" and not attacking it.

There are two primary attributes of stem cells that make them so exciting as potential treatments through transplantation. First, they are undifferentiated cells that have not yet formed a particular function and usually only do so when they mature in specific parts of the body. Second, unlike mature cells in various parts of the body, stem cells are self-replicating, meaning that they can divide and replicate many times over. As a result, scientists can grow these cells in the laboratory until they have literally millions of cells for study and for potential use in therapies.

Not all stem cells, however, are the same. Embryonic stem cells come from embryos and are totipotent in the early stages after fertilization. This means that these cells have the ability to turn into any kind of cell, including a host of embryonic cells needed to form a human, such as placenta cells. After several days following conception, these cells become pluripotent. They can form into any kind of cell found in an adult but not the variety of cells that form an embryo. As a result, these cells become the various and multiple specialized cells that form the heart, lung, skin, and other tissues in the human body.

Adult stem cells are found in the body after birth and are in general multipotent cells, meaning that they create the types of tissues in which they are found, such as those found in the bone marrow for creating the various types of blood cells. These cells are found in organs and tissues throughout the body, including the brain, blood vessels, liver, and muscles, and are believed to remain there undivided until they are needed to create new cells following damage, such as disease or injury. However, research over the last several years indicates that the stem cells found in one part of the body may also have the ability to form specific cells found in other parts of the body, which is known as plasticity. For example, some studies have shown that hematopoietic (blood-forming) stem cells can develop into heart muscle.

Stem cell transplantation is still in the early stages and has many hurdles to overcome. A significant ethical debate (discussed in Chapter 9) has arisen over the use of embryonic stem cells, which researchers acquire from human embryos developed from eggs fertilized in vitro (outside of the woman's body). These cells that are developed for in vitro fertilization clinics are donated for research when they are not used and have been approved for research use by the donors. Because research with these cells is still in its early stages, scientists are not sure how the cells will react once placed inside the human body. For example, they could proliferate too much and "overgrow," which occurs with cancer cells. There is also the question of immunity and rejection by the transplant recipient. In 2001 President George W. Bush set legal limitations to research with embryonic stem cells in the United States. He gave an executive order that federally funded research could only use existing embryonic stem cell lines, which limits the number of stem cells available for these researchers. Although seventeen new stem cell lines were created in March 2003 from private funds, any researcher funded by government monies is banned from using these cells. (See Annotated Primary Documents.)

Most scientists consider these embryonic cells as the most promising stem cells for therapeutic use. Although adult stem cells have therapeutic potential, they appear to be much more limited than embryonic stem cells in their ability to differentiate. They also are not readily available in great numbers, can be hard to find and extract, and are more difficult to proliferate in the laboratory setting.

Although many scientists believe effective therapies developed from stem cells are many years away, a group of scientists at Stanford University Medical Center received approval from the U.S. Food and Drug Administration in October 2005 to transplant stem cells into the brains of six children suffering from Batten disease. This rare, degenerative, and fatal genetic disorder first causes its victims to go blind and then to lose speech and ultimately become paralyzed before dying. The fetal stem cells used in the Stanford therapy are not embryonic stem cells but rather immature neural cells that will ultimately develop into the variety of fully grown cells that make the brain. Scientists hope that these cells will form an essential enzyme that is missing in these patients and needed to dispose of neural cellular waste.

HAND TRANSPLANTS

Although organ transplants may now seem commonplace, limb transplantation has largely remained the fancy of science fiction writers. In 1964 a hand transplant was attempted in South America, but the recipient's immune system rejected the transplant within two weeks. The surgery was essentially shelved until organ-transplant specialists developed effective immunosuppressive drug regimens. Then, in 1998, surgeons in Lyon, France, performed a successful hand transplant on New Zealand man. Since that time, more than twenty-five hand transplants have been completed.

The procedure is complex and difficult. It includes bone fixation and repair and attachment of tendons, arteries, nerves, and veins. To illustrate just how arduous the surgery is, a typical heart transplant takes six to eight hours whereas a hand transplant usually takes from eight to twelve hours.

Although hand transplants obtained from a cadaveric donor can enhance both the function and the appearance of patients, there are many issues to consider with this surgery. Just like with organ transplants, hand transplant recipients must undergo a considerable, ongoing regimen of immunosuppression, which has unknown long-term risks. The patient also risks acute rejection and infection from opportunistic organisms. Some surgeons question whether a patient should undergo such significant risks in a procedure that is not necessary for saving a patient's life.

There are also psychological issues to consider. Unlike organ transplants, the transplanted hand is continuously visible. For example, the New Zealand man who received a transplanted hand later requested that it be amputated, which doctors did a little more than two years after the initial operation. Doctors noted that the man did not follow the immunosuppressive regiment assigned to him, leading his body to reject the transplanted hand. The man, however, complained that the transplanted hand felt like a dead person's hand that had no feeling. He was quoted as saying he felt "mentally detached" from the transplanted hand (BBC News Online, 2001).

Ethical concerns about transplanted hands include the ability of the patient to thoroughly understand the risks and make good judgments about following the drug regimen properly and exercising the hand. Another concern is whether the patient's improved quality of life is commensurate with the potential hazards involved. Some observers worry that the time and effort put into the procedure by the doctors and the emotional demands on the patient may make both the doctors and the patients less willing to amputate the hand if something goes wrong. For example, in the case of the New Zealand patient, both the patient and his doctors struggled over whether to remove the transplanted hand for many months before it was finally amputated. The psychological challenges to a hand-transplant recipient may also be special in some ways. Unlike transplanted organs, a hand from a deceased donor is always visible, which could have an uncomfortable psychological impact. In the final analysis, although acceptable functional and cosmetic outcomes have been achieved with hand transplants, it remains an experimental procedure that requires much further research.

FACE TRANSPLANTS

The possibility of transplanting a face became much more than just a theoretical dream following the successful transplantation of hands in the late 1990s. Bolstered by advances in hand transplantation, which included refined microsurgical techniques, surgeons began to openly state that a face transplant would be performed in the not-too-distant future. They were right. On November 27, 2005, surgeons in Amiens, France, completed a partial face transplant on a woman who had been disfigured by her dog several months earlier.

The process involved removal of a brain-dead donor's face, which was then chilled in a saline solution at 29 degrees Fahrenheit for transportation. (A silicone prosthesis was made from a cast of the donor's face and used for viewing the deceased.) Attaching the facial parts involved grafting the nose, lips, and chin from the donor with microsurgical techniques similar to those used in hand-transplant surgeries. Next, surgeons connected the blood vessels to the face, and blood flow was successfully restored within four hours after the face had been removed from the donor. Finally, surgeons connected the numerous facial muscles and nerves, which the head surgeon, Jean-Michel Dubernard, described as being "as fine as the fibers hanging from a string bean" (Smith, *New York Times*, 2005). The operation took fifteen hours to complete, and Dubernard later injected stem cells from the donor's bone marrow in an effort to improve the ability of the patient's immune system to accept the graft.

Within a week, the recipient, a thirty-nine-year-old French woman named Isabelle Dinoire, was eating and drinking and able to talk clearly. The only sign of the surgery was a thin scar around the transplanted area. Almost three months later, Dinoire was making remarkable strides, including a return of sensation to the transplanted areas. Several surgical teams in the United Sates, France, and the Netherlands also announced that they would attempt a face transplant, including an entire face transplant. Even with a complete face transplant, however, recipients will not look like the donor. Most experts believe the person will look entirely different but may retain some semblance of their former selves because the donor face is grafted onto the recipient's existing bone and muscle. Furthermore, facial mannerisms such as squinting and blushing may remain similar because they are hardwired in the brain and have less to do with facial structure.

Face transplants became controversial when they were first proposed, and the debate has not gone away following the first successful transplant. Much like hand transplants, face transplants represent high risks for rejection and infections, which leads to the same argument that such potentially fatal risks should not be attempted unless they are a matter of life and death. The psychological impact could also be tremendous, especially if the face is ultimately rejected by the immune system and has to be removed. However, proponents argue that these surgeries are not just cosmetic procedures but can provide a new life for people who have suffered severe disfigurement resulting from a variety of causes, such as burns and shootings.

THE FUTURE OF TRANSPLANTATION

This chapter has covered only the most highly touted advances in transplantation. New research protocols both within and outside of the field promise to propel transplantation even further. For example, there have been efforts to expand organ availability by enabling transplant candidates to receive kidneys from live donors with traditionally incompatible blood types through a protocol consisting of spleen removal, medications, and a type of blood filtering called plasmapheresis.

Technological advances such as laparoscopic surgery have made removing kidneys from a live donor less invasive and, in the process, have increased the safety and likelihood of finding such donors. For example, in 2003 the number of kidneys transplanted from live donors outnumbered deceased donor rates for the first time.

Numerous areas of research are underway to further advance transplantation. For example, researchers at Carnegie Mellon University are investigating the use of magnetic resonance imaging (MRI) to track immune cells as they infiltrate a transplanted heart in the early stages of organ rejection. If ultimately successful, the technology could be used to detect rejection earlier than ever before, allowing the medical team to better manage patients and save more lives.

Many debates have arisen over transplantation during the past five decades. Some have been addressed, but few have been resolved conclusively. Modern advances and the rapid rise of technology have brought about new questions as well. The following chapters focus on some of the most pressing and hotly debated issues in transplantation and transplantation-related areas. Issues such as the equitable allocation of donor organs, selling organs, and replacing human organs and other body parts with those of animals will not be easily resolved.

SECTION TWO

Controversies and Issues Relating to Transplantation

CHAPTER 5

Buying and Selling Organs for Donation

The lack of donor organs may be the single most important issue in transplantation. Established as an effective, lifesaving therapy, transplantation has advanced by the proverbial "leaps and bounds." Most experts agree that the science, in essence, will take care of itself as new drugs, technologies, and research discoveries ensure a bright future.

Acquiring enough donor organs, however, has remained an unrealized goal and has led to thousands of deaths in the United States and many more globally. Despite efforts to increase public education and awareness of the need coupled with legislation to improve request-for-donation procedures and performance—thousands of patients on the transplant waiting list die each year because a donor organ is not available. One approach to solving the problems is xenotransplantation, or the use of animal organs such as those of pigs. Although highly promising, current research is at the basic science level, and xenotransplantation is likely many years away from becoming an alternative source of organs.

The use of live donors when possible, such as in the case of some kidney and liver transplants, has increased significantly in response to organ shortages and to improved patient care that lessens risk to the donor. Few would argue, however, that live donation is the answer to the problem. First of all, it's not viable for some transplants, such as the heart. Second, if people are not willing to donate their organs after they die, how much more difficult would it be to convince people to donate organs when they are still alive, especially considering the potential risks associated with any invasive surgery? As a result, most live donors are socially connected to the transplant recipient in some way, such as family, friends, or members of a church group.

Selling Prisoners' Organs

Despite banning its own hospitals from partaking in the practice after an international outcry, China's Health Ministry has looked the other way regarding the continued sale of executed prisoners' organs for transplantation. Chinese officials have admitted that through their military hospitals they have sold prisoners' organs to foreign transplant recipients. For example, a liver is reportedly sold for around $20,000 to a foreign recipient and perhaps for as high as $41,000 dollars to a recipient from the West.

The practice has raised strong objections from human rights activists around the world. As a country, China executes 15,000 prisoners each year, which is more than all other judicial executions in the world combined. With concerns already raised over China's likelihood to protect their prisoners' individual rights or guarantee due process in a criminal trial, critics argue that taking organs from prisoners for financial gain would increase pressure for conviction and execution.

In a 2001 Washington hearing, then Assistant Secretary of State Michael E. Parmly testified that unconfirmed reports have pointed to the removal of organs from living prisoners. Parmly noted, "We consider organ harvesting from executed prisoners, without permission from family members, to be an egregious human rights abuse that violates not only international human rights law, but also international medical ethical standards" (Parmly, 2001). In 2005 China's Ministry of Health announced that it was establishing laws to completely ban the sale of human organs and to develop stricter overall transplant regulations and operations.

A highly controversial proposal to solving the organ shortage problem is to provide financial incentives or establish a market system for purchasing human organs. Proponents of these approaches believe that financial incentives will lead to higher organ-donation rates at levels that can solve the organ shortage problem. They also believe that a market-system approach can be conducted ethically with safeguards for fair management and to avoid abuse.

Opponents to financial incentives counter that embarking on such a policy to increase organ donation is a slippery slope involving many ethical dilemmas. They fear exploitation of the poor and an unfair advantage to procure lifesaving organs going to the rich. Concerns have also arisen about how financial incentives might affect the doctor–patient relationship, moving the patient into the realm of both commodity and consumer. In addition, some countries, such as China, have already admitted to being involved in an international black market for organs (see sidebar.)

This chapter examines arguments on both sides of the issues concerning the sale of human organs. With advancing science and technology, our bodies can be viewed physically as intricate biological machines with replaceable parts. On the other hand, our notion of ourselves and the value we place on our body have placed deeply ingrained societal, religious, and psychological boundaries on what we can or perhaps should do with our bodies.

MORE THAN A BODY

The idea of the human body as a sacred temple that houses our mind, and thus is deserving of respect, dates back to ancient societies and religions, which helped establish beliefs and rituals to care for the body after death. Another example of our "reverence" for the human body is the taboo placed on suicide within most cultures. When accepted, suicide is usually a highly ritualized process, such as the well-known ritual of Hara-Kari once practiced in Japan. Japanese warriors and military men, for example, were sanctioned and encouraged by their leaders and the state to disembowel themselves rather than disgrace their country with defeat, capture, and coming home to remind everyone of "losing face." Ironically, the value placed on the human body is also represented by those ancient civilizations that conducted ritualistic human sacrifices. In their minds, only a human, both in spirit and body, could appease the gods.

Ritualistic suicide and human sacrifice exist only as aberrations in modern society, but we have maintained the idea of the sacredness of the body. Human parts such as the heart have become symbolic within our deepest psyche, and they probably never will be thought of in strictly scientific terms. These notions play a fundamental role in many medical controversies, including the marketing of organs and the controversy over stem cell transplants (see Chapter 9). Although most modern societies and their religious institutions have approved organ donation and recognized it as an act of love, charity, and even duty, the idea of "selling" lifesaving organs has for the most part remained outside the realm of legitimacy. For example, in an address to a transplant conference, Pope John Paul II noted,

> The human body is always a personal body, the body of a person. The body cannot be treated as a merely physical or biological entity, nor can its organs and tissues ever be used as items for sale or exchange. Such a reductive materialist conception would lead to a merely instrumental use of the

body, and therefore of the person. In such a perspective, organ transplantation and the grafting of tissue would no longer correspond to an act of donation but would amount to the dispossession or plundering of a body. (O'Rourke and Boyle, 1993, p. 221)

Nevertheless, some ethicists and various groups have come to believe that the sale of human organs is ethical. Even religious organizations have approved at one time or another. For example, the Ad Hoc Administration of the Ministry of Waqfs [religious endowments] and Islamic Affairs passed a fatwa (a ruling on a point of Islamic law given by a recognized authority) in the 1980s that read,

> As for the patient's purchase of a kidney from another person, the rule is that such act is impermissible, because Allah has honoured man, so it is not permitted to cut some of his organs and sell them at any price, whatsoever, but if the patient does not find a donor to give him his kidney, and his life is endangered, while he cannot find any other means to cure his illness, then purchase of organs is permissible, because the patient, then, is driven by a dire necessity. (Abul-Fotouh, 1987)

It is this "dire necessity" that is driving the debate over whether human organs should be bought and sold or whether some other financially based incentives should be used to increase donation. On a fundamental psychological level, the idea of selling organs is an aberration and desecration, like old horror movies in which bodies were dug up for medical research. Proponents of organ sales say we must move beyond these "instincts" and point out that the current system has never effectively supplied enough organs to save the lives of a great many of those who have needed them.

THE PUBLIC POLICY

More than 90,784 people were on the organ transplant waiting list as of early 2005, which is nearly a threefold increase of the 31,000 patients on the waiting list in 1992. In 2004 an average of eighteen men, women, and children died each day waiting for an organ transplant, for a total of 6,529 people over the course of the year. However, some observers believe that these statistics belie the actual number of people who die each year because donor organs are not found in time to save their lives. For example, patients are removed from the list when they become too sick while waiting for an organ and, as a result, are not healthy enough to receive a transplant. Many, if not most, of these people die from their illnesses but are not a part of the official statistics. Furthermore, observers argue that many people whose lives could be saved by a transplant never reach the waiting list because shortages have made getting a transplant a more stringent process. As a result, these patients are unlikely to get an organ because of any number of criteria, including age and chance of long-term survival.

Practically speaking, concerns over the sale of humans' organs began in the early 1980s when markets began to appear for human kidneys harvested from live donors. As a result, the U.S. National Organ Transplant Act of 1984 included a provision that outlawed payment for individual's providing organs for transplantation. The act states, "It shall be unlawful for any person to knowingly acquire, receive or otherwise transfer any human organ for valuable consideration for use in human transplantation" (Reams, 1984). As a result, no money or valuable property has been allowed to pass among donor, recipient, and organ broker in the procurement of donor organs in the United States for more than two decades. Although the initiative for the provision was to prevent living donors from selling their organs to the highest bidders, the act also prevents people from selling the right to harvest their organs after they died.

This view of "no-sale" when it comes to procuring organs is largely but not completely shared worldwide. For example, the World Health Organization (WHO) has declared that the commercialization of human organs is "a violation of human rights" and "human dignity." Primarily concerned with commercial trafficking of living donor organs, the WHO established the following principal: "The human body and its parts cannot be the subject of commercial transactions. Accordingly, giving or receiving payment (including any other compensation or reward) for organs should be prohibited" (World Health Organization, 1991).

Despite such proclamations, few, if any, people would dispute the fact that the current system based on altruism does not work in terms of supplying enough organs or, to take a more economic view, fulfilling market demand. Efforts such as public education to foster altruistic donations have increased organ recovery by 15 percent. Nevertheless, although a national average of 45 percent of people consent to become organ donors, demand far outstrips supply. In fact, a vast difference exists in the number of those who consent to organ donation upon death and the number of organs that are actually harvested and suitable for transplantation. For example, improved trauma efforts have resulted in a reduction in accidental deaths where "healthy" organs can be retrieved. In the end, although Americans generally agree that organ donation is a laudable contribution to society, the majority of them do not live up to the ideal.

The discussion about the use of money or other incentives to purchase organs for transplantation has gone on for many years. However, more ethicists and health professionals are beginning to seriously consider the potential to solve the organ-shortage problem by buying and selling organs. This discussion reflects partly on the many successes and the growth in transplantation. Nevertheless, as noted in the *American Transplant Journal* by authors Jeffrey P. Kahn and Francis L. Delmonico, "The consideration of payments for live vendors by physicians is placing the transplant community at an ethical and professional crossroad that is a departure from the standard of the past fifty years" (Kahn and Delmonico, 2004, p. 178).

THE PROPOSALS

Writing in the *George Mason Law Review*, Steve P. Calandrillo succinctly stated the case for the exploration of potentially establishing an economically based organ market when he noted, "Since thousands die each year while waiting for organs that never arrive, we must explore incentives that can change this terrible outcome" (Calandrillo, 2004, p. 69). The ideas for the "buying and selling" of organs are varied but can basically be broken down into two categories: developing regulated markets in organ sales or creating other types of incentives and rewards to boost donation rates.

THE INCENTIVE APPROACH

The incentive approach to procuring more donor organs seeks to avoid direct monetary payment for organs. In essence, it is making a distinction between "incentives" and "payments." As noted in a report by the Payment Subcommittee of the UNOS Ethics Committee, "A system of financial incentives may indeed be a viable option if, as interpreted by law, 'incentives' do not amount to 'purchases' and 'donors' are therefore not transformed into 'vendors'" (UNOS Sharing Ethics Committee Payment Subcommittee, 1993).

Although this consideration may sound like an exercise in semantics, it is important because it largely seeks to avoid direct monetary enrichment and the potential pitfalls associated with it, such as the exploitation of poor people to sell their organs without taking into serious consideration the health risks or without their receiving their fair share financially for the transaction. Organizations such as the American Medical Association, the United Network for Organ Sharing (UNOS), and the American Society of Transplant Surgeons have explored the issue of incentives. In recent years Congress has debated several bills addressing the issue in various ways, including reimbursement of medical and nonmedical expenses for qualifying donors.

Incentives to become an organ donor are wide-ranging and generally seek to increase people's inclination to sign up and become an organ donor. For example, there is the relatively simple offer of providing driver's license discounts to people who agree to become organ donors in case of their death. The state of Georgia, for example, offers a reduced fee for driver's license renewal if the individual chooses to be an organ donor. Another approach in terms of reward is the idea of income tax or estate benefits, which has been considered by Congress. Other incentive-based ideas include reimbursement for the funeral expenses of donors or a charitable contribution to an organization named by the deceased or the family.

An additional approach that avoids the direct exchange of currency is the idea of "paired organ exchanges." The concept revolves around the notion that many relatives may be willing to donate a live kidney or to become a live donor, for example, for a family member who needs an organ to save his or her life. However, family members may not be compatible donors because of tissue type or other biological factors. In this approach, these people would be able to arrange a paired organ exchange with family members from another patient needing a transplant and who are compatible with the opposing family member. A variation of this idea is to expand the program even further by providing the incentive of moving a family member higher up the waiting list if another family member becomes a living donor for anyone else. A nonprofit voluntary network of organ donors called LifeSharers has already established a related approach. Members of the program agree to donate their organs after they die and, in return, are given first access to other fellow members' organs. While many perceive this as a "fair" approach that gives priority to people willing to donate their own organs, others point out that the approach is still discriminatory to those who cannot donate for various personal reasons, such as personal finances or religion, and who thus would be at a disadvantage in obtaining an organ because they cannot join the program. Critics also point out that such an organization's membership might not grow large enough to supply organs when needed.

THE MARKET-BASED APPROACH

Although debates do surround various notions of "indirect" incentives for becoming an organ donor, developing a regulated market for the financial procurement of organs is by far the most contentious proposal on the table, seen by critics as being a situation ripe for abuse. Nevertheless, economists, lawyers, ethicists, physicians, and others have laid out serious proposals for a market-based approach to transplantation.

One inventive approach is to establish a "futures market" in transplantation in which people are paid for the right to harvest their organs after they die, like a futures contract in investing. If a viable organ is harvested when the person dies, the deceased's named beneficiary would receive payment. This approach is preferred by some to immediate payment because it potentially would help avoid exploiting the poor by prohibiting live donor sales. A variation of this proposal has the potential donor receiving reduced insurance rates for agreeing to donate at death.

Another "commodities" approach is the "spot market" approach, in which family members are approached about the sale of the deceased's organs. The American Society of Transplant Surgeons' Ad Hoc Committee to End the Intractable Shortage of Human Organs examined the issue of providing direct payment to the family estate through what it deems an acceptable form, such as a charitable donation. A member of the committee, Alexander Tabarrok, who has also served as an associate professor of economics at George Mason University, has commented that some believe a direct money payment would also be appropriate to the deceased's estate as a kind of "thank you" for the donation. Tabarrok noted that the committee developed language for approaching families on the spot and informing them of an incentive-based plan for organ donation with the incentives going to the estate of the donor. The text would read something like this:

> Dear Mr. Smith/Ms. Jones, as you may know, it is our standard policy to offer a gift of $5,000 to the estate of the deceased, as a way of saying "Thank you for giving the gift of life." The money can be used to help offset funeral or hospital expenses, to donate to your loved one's favorite charity, or simply to remain with the estate, to be used in any manner the heirs see fit. No price can be placed upon the many lives that can be saved by your gift. Our donation in return is merely society's way of honoring the sacrifice you are being asked to make, and is a token of our deep and sincere appreciation for your generosity at this most difficult time. (Tabarrok, 2004)

Once again, semantics comes into play, but a direct, hard-core market approach would likely be based on market-determined prices that would fluctuate. In their book *The U.S. Organ Procurement System, A Prescription for Reform*, David L. Kaserman and A.H. Barnett outline how such a system might work. After acquiring the organ, the organ procurement firm would sell it to a transplant center, which would in turn include the costs on its bills at the exact price paid to the donor or donor's estate. The organs would be allocated in the same manner under UNOS laws. The extra expenses incurred for purchasing the organ could be paid for by insurance, transplant groups, government sources, or the transplant recipient.

Some market-based proposals also include the idea of a living-donor organ market, despite its significant potential for abuse, such as black markets. Of course, the question arises about the "going price" for an organ. Investigators at the University of Buffalo estimated that the price for a kidney in 2006 would be approximately $15,000, and the price for a liver would be as high as $35,000. Others have estimated the market-clearing price to be about $5,000 for a kidney. The fact is that no one can be sure of how supply and demand would affect prices in a highly regulated market.

THE GOVERNMENT AND THE SANCTITY OF THE HUMAN BODY

The debate surrounding the sale of human organs revolves around two primary considerations. The first states that the sale of human organs goes against human dignity. The second argues that a market-based approach would be inequitable.

The immorality of commodifying the human body is deeply ingrained in most societies. In the United States, for example, government bodies long ago established that our body's sanctity is an inalienable right in terms of autonomy and dignity. Furthermore, prevailing morality and law have rejected the view that we are free to do whatever we wish with our bodies. Examples include morally based bans on such things as prostitution, drug abuse, and incest. The ban against selling organ falls within this purview.

Those who favor organ sales have argued that moral objections "reflect a state of moral paternalism rather than pragmatism" (Kishore, *Journal of Medical Ethics*, 2005, p. 362). Even if the moral basis were appropriate, they contend that the government is contradicting itself by taking a moral stand that purchasing human body parts is wrong, considering that human tissues and products arc already part of a thriving market, such as profit-making sperm and ova fertility banks.

Those on the other side of the philosophical fence, however, have argued that there is a significant difference between selling regenerative body parts such as sperm and selling nonregenerative organs that are the very basis of life. Furthermore, they argue, selling organs is a step in making a commodity out of life itself. Not only would this have a psychological impact of debasing our views of ourselves, but it would also lead to concrete, real-life problems and abuses.

EXPLOITING THE POOR

A logical and often-used argument against buying and selling live donor organs is that establishing a payment system for organs arbitrarily assigns to body parts market values that involve gender, ethnicity, and social status factors. The primary concern is that the rich would benefit immensely from such a system at both the financial and physical expense of the poorer segments of society.

Opponents to a market system contend that poorer people might act impulsively out of financial needs and not fully consider the potential medical risks. They also note that people who are financially secure would be less likely to donate in such a system, and the poor would become the major source of live donor organs and, as a result, would take on the predominant burden of risk. The first risk lies with the operation itself, such as the donor developing bleeding or infections or suffering from an injured spleen. There may also be long-term risks. For example, although no increased risk for developing kidney failure is apparent in donors, individuals left with one kidney have a slightly higher incidence of developing high blood pressure.

A libertarian approach to the problem favors organ sales, noting that in a free society people should have the freedom to address their problems in the best way they can as long as it is not illegal. If they can improve their situation in life by selling their organs, they should be allowed to do so. Opponents are concerned, however, that selling organs could result in various segments of our society creating incentives for reducing options for the poor to better themselves, thus making their likelihood to donate organs greater.

Perhaps the biggest argument against the sale of organs is that it may ultimately not help the poor very much at all. Reports from the sale of organs in India indicate that it has negatively impacted the poor sellers medically, socially, and at times even financially. According to a 2002 study, approximately 350 people who were interviewed received a little more than $1,000 for a kidney. Most of the donors later reported that they sold the kidney to address debts, but almost three-quarters of them reported still being in debt six years later. Furthermore, more than 85 percent reported a decline in health after their donation, and nearly 80 percent said they would not recommend others to sell a kidney.

Pakistan has also experienced an unregulated and fast-growing kidney transplant trade based on foreign purchasers. Payments to the donor could range widely but normally fell within the $1,000 to $4,000 dollar range. Granted, this is a significant amount of money for a poor Pakistani, but nevertheless, after paying off debts and other costs, the donors could end up

---

Come and Get Them

Pakistan's reputation as a place favorable to "transplant tourism" is well known, with newspapers carrying small ads and private hospitals even advertising their services on the Internet. Nevertheless, Thor Andersen, a London-based millionaire, made news when he bought a kidney from a Pakistani girl named Sumaira in 2002 and then filed an insurance claim for the organ purchase and surgical procedure. Andersen argued that it would have cost his insurance company far more money to keep him on dialysis. Although he was on a transplant waiting list in Great Britain, Andersen feared that an organ would not arrive in time to save his life. His twenty-two-year-old donor was from Punjab province, a place noted for its trade in living donors. Although she and her family received $3,200 for the kidney, they ultimately went home with around $750 after repaying loans and other debts, the broker, and postoperative care costs.

---

with as little as several hundred dollars in many instances. In 2006 the Pakistani government announced that it was preparing to ban transplant "tourism." (See sidebar.)

Opponents further argue that abuses in places such as India and Pakistan would also occur in an unfettered market-based system for live organ donations. In their *American Journal of Transplantation* article, Kahn and Delmonico wrote,

> Our view is that policies that allow the selling of organs represent a failure themselves. They signal a willingness to accept a policy environment that would make exploitation of the worst off a societal-endorsed rule rather than the exception to be prevented. Moreover, government sanction of organ sales would represent an undermining of a moral foundation of our society that views government as having responsibility to provide for the poor. (Kahn and Delmonico, *American Journal of Transplantation*, 2004)

Proponents of the market system believe that tight government control of markets would reduce and practically eliminate abuses and efforts at coercion:

> Under the current system, a physician, nurse, or organ procurement officer must try to coax the family of the deceased to give away for free an asset that could be worth several hundred dollars. Which system involves greater coercion? By favoring the current altruistic system over the market system, the

proponent is merely substituting moral or emotional coercion for the alleged "economic coercion" that would accompany a market system. (Kaserman and Barnett, *The U.S. Organ Procurement System: A Prescription for Reform*, 2002, p. 77)

Proponents further contend that insurance and government funding, such as vouchers based on income to help level the playing field, could counterbalance the unfair advantage that goes to the rich in a paying system. Nevertheless, government regulations are not guarantees against abuses. Furthermore, some argue that it would be wrong to limit transactions to government-regulated markets. Why not solve the organ-shortage problem and get a better price through other market-based systems, such as bartering on the Internet? (See sidebar.)

One approach to solving the socioeconomic discrepancies and biases inherent in a market-based system of organ procurement is to develop a commercial system with an altruistic component. For example, a voluntary organ-donation system could also be maintained in which the organs provided through this system would be earmarked primarily for the poor whereas people with enough money or adequate insurance coverage would still purchase an organ. Some opponents believe that even this system would ultimately have a negative impact on the poor because the majority of people would opt to sell their organs, thus lowering the number of organs donated for altruistic reasons and reducing the number of organs available for the poor. There are also concerns that these organs would be of a lower quality.

Proponents of this combined commercial-altruistic system counter that strict government oversight could protect against abuses. They point out that a quota could be placed on how many organs can be supplied within the system by people at low-income levels. They also believe that organs might not come primarily from the poor, especially in the case of living donations because many family members would still continue to donate. Furthermore, proponents contend that the higher rate of diseases and organ damage resulting from drug use or other problems, which are statistically more prevalent in the poor, would make many of them unsuitable as organ donors.

Although much of the debate concerning exploitation of the poor has focused on live donations, opponents of using market-system approaches to increase organ donation rates also believe that cadaveric donations for profit would also adversely affect this segment of the population. In addition to the issues already raised about some people's ability to "afford" an organ, they suggest that poor people might sign irrevocable contracts, would not be able to buy their way out of such contracts, and still would not be able to afford to purchase an organ if they needed one.

BLACK MARKETS

There is little doubt that black markets exist for transplant organs or that they profit from "transplant tourism," in which wealthy patients seek out live donors primarily in underdeveloped countries or locales. In December 2003, South African and Brazilian police captured the leaders

---

Internet Brokering for Organs

The idea sounds like a good one. New Internet clearinghouses have been established to connect organ-transplant recipients with altruistic strangers willing to donate organs. The first donor organ procured through a Web site was transplanted on October 20, 2004, at Presbyterian/St. Luke's Medical Center in Denver, Colorado. The thirty-two-year-old donor, named Robert Smitty, responded to an ad from a fifty-eight-year-old physician named Bob Hickey, who advertised on the MatchingDonors.com Web site for a membership fee of $295 per month. The donor noted that he chose to donate a kidney to Dr. Hickey because the ill physician had a family, including a wife and two sons.

Designated live-organ donation has long been accepted, but most cases involve relatives and friends who are seeking to save a loved one's life. Critics of Internet brokering, however, note several problems, including adhering to the altruistic notion of organ donation. They argue that strict oversight would be needed to make sure that individuals are not being paid for their organs. For example, Hickey did pay Smitty around $5,000 as allowed by law to cover the trip to Denver and other expenses. Other problems noted include inequality in distribution and potential extortion. Abuses could also occur in terms of the donor providing accurate medical data and reports on personal behaviors. The argument was summed up by United Network for Organ Sharing (UNOS) official Joel Newman, who noted,

> Transplant candidates certainly can exercise free speech and talk about their specific need. However, transplant professionals are concerned with the concept of a service that allows some candidates to purchase more public exposure of their need, where others lack the knowledge or means to do so. Any perceived favoritism or differential treatment could weaken public trust and potentially make people less willing to become donors, which would hurt all transplant patients. (Barclay, Medscape Medical News, 2004)

of an international ring trafficking in human kidneys. A village in India, which banned kidney sales in 1994, is referred to locally as "kidney village" because so many residents have illegally sold one of their kidneys for transplantation, perhaps for as little as a few hundred dollars. Prior to invasion by the United States in 2003, Iraq had a sophisticated black-market operation in human organs. Other countries such as Israel, Turkey, Russia, Argentina, and Brazil are also known not to stringently enforce their laws prohibiting human organ sale and purchases.

Some argue that the black market in illegal organ transplants also leads to "illegal" transplants in the United States. According to Calandrillo, "There is no national transplant screening board in the United States; each hospital sets its own rules for who can be a live organ donor. Foreign patients often arrive with a willing, unrelated 'donor' and money in hand. Some U.S. hospitals have a 'don't ask, don't tell' policy with respect to foreigner organ transplants, and organ brokers know how to find these hospitals" (Calandrillo, *George Mason Law Review*, 2004).

Opponents to the sale of organs believe that legitimizing their sale could result in the growth of black markets by increasing the overall economic market for organ sales. Proponents counter that a legally regulated organ marketplace, both for deceased and living donors, would increase the supply of legal donors and reduce the need for wealthy foreigners to partake in organ tourism. Even if the organs could be obtained cheaper on the black market, they believe most people would choose the regulated market because of insurance of better-quality organs than on the black market, where people, in order to make money, may hide health problems that could impact the organ's condition.

SOCIETAL COSTS OF A MARKET SYSTEM

Whether it is the direct sale of organs or some type of incentive program, opponents believe that the increased control of the process by the government and private organ brokers could result in a significantly heavier burden on society because of administrative costs and other requirements needed to implement and run the system. Furthermore, they argue that society will also have to maintain the burden of costs for those live donors whose health may decline because of the donation.

One answer to the latter problem, according to proponents of selling organs, is to establish an insurance fund to which organ sellers are required to contribute from the money they make selling their organs. They compare this approach to liability insurance required for risky behaviors such as driving or performing certain occupations.

As for administrative and other costs incurred by society, proponents of sales and incentives for organ donors note that there are already hefty administrative costs in the current system that get passed on one way or another to the health care consumer or insurance company. In terms of government expenditures, the Bush administration's 2006 budget proposal included $22,282,000 earmarked for government running and oversight of transplant operations, including operation of OPTN and the Scientific Registry of Transplant Recipients, educational efforts to raise the number of organ donors, and a demonstration project grant for the reimbursement of travel and subsistence expenses towards living organ donation.

Those in favor of marketing organs claim that a market system will ultimately save money. For example, studies have shown that kidney transplants are cheaper than patients receiving dialysis over a lifetime and that, when compared to dialysis, kidney transplants essentially pay for themselves within a couple of years. Furthermore, the federal government's End Stage Renal Disease (ESRD) program pays for the majority of costs associated with dialysis, costs that could be greatly reduced. It has been estimated that each live kidney donor saves the federal government approximately $94,576 per patient (Matas and Schnitzler, *American Journal of Transplantation*, 2004). Estimates on what the government could actually save through a market-based kidney donor program range from $30 to $200 million a year.

Another financial issue associated with costs concerns the question of who benefits financially from the current altruistic system of organ procurement and allocation. Costs for a transplant vary according to factors such as where the operation is performed and the development of complications, which leads to longer hospital stays and higher expenses. Nevertheless, according to estimates made by the National Foundation for Transplants, these are the typical costs, minus pre- or posttransplant treatments:

- Bone Marrow—$250,000
- Heart—$300,000
- Heart/Lung—$300,000 to $350,000
- Isolated Small Bowel—$350,000
- Kidney—$75,000 to $100,000
- Kidney/Pancreas—$150,000
- Liver—$250,000
- Lung—$200,000 to $250,000
- Pancreas—$100,000

Proponents of buying and selling organs believe that it is inherently unfair that surgeons, hospitals, organ brokers, and many others involved in the "business" of organ transplantation make money while the donors or their families receive no benefit other than those personal benefits associated with altruism. Another view is that donor rates would increase if donors and families were paid for organs because it would place organ donation more in the guise of a social obligation rather than a difficult moral decision that some people might not want to make. However, according to anecdotal reports, families of organ donors have also indicated that the offer of a "financial incentive" for donation would have been perceived as coercion and might have changed their decision to donate.

THE ONGOING DEBATE

Much of the debate around incentives and markets for buying and selling organs is based on anecdotal evidence and personal belief. Proponents of these approaches believe that they are on solid ethical ground, arguing that the system would be based on concern for patients and saving lives. Opponents counter that the altruistic system has not failed and just needs to be better promoted through education and training programs.

For now, little data is available to shed light on whether various organ-market policies would increase the supply of organs. Proponents, established medical institutions, and even some in government are calling for "demonstration" projects to research the feasibility of marketing organs or providing various incentives for donation to increase donor organ supplies. Ultimately, however, the answer to this issue probably will not lie in statistics alone but rather will incorporate many moral judgments concerning more exact definitions of personal dignity and the nobility of the medical profession. Regardless, the issue remains that people are dying because of a lack of donor organs.

CHAPTER 6

Organ Allocation: Who Should Get an Organ?

Controversy will surround the issue of organ allocation as long as not enough donor organs are available for all the patients who need them. Although organ donation rates have slowly risen, these rates are unable to keep up with demand, and the organ-donor shortage grows larger every year. With approximately seventeen to eighteen patients dying each day because an organ is not available for them, many questions about organ allocation continue to plague the field of transplantation, despite the many rules and regulations regarding allocation and their changes over the years (see Chapter 3).

Although the approximately 6,200 or so deaths per year of patients waiting for an organ transplant are just a tiny fraction of the overall mortality rate in the United States, the causes of these deaths are easily identifiable, and the deaths are generally considered preventable. As a result, they have a high amount of visibility in the general public and carry with them political and social significance. For the most part, the U.S. public has generally accepted the current organ-allocation system as medically justifiable and defensible on moral grounds. This belief is based on the assumption that the current policies are the best achievable ones for balancing the principles of utility (that is, making the best use of available organs) and equity (that is, providing organs in a fair manner). Nevertheless, as transplant professionals achieve greater success rates in terms of prolonging and improving quality of life and in providing transplants to a wider variety of patients, the growing demand for transplantation is placing the allocation system under increasing scrutiny.

Many questions continue to surround organ-allocation policies. In dealing with such a valuable and limited resource, should patients who are the sickest get a transplant instead of a healthier patient with a better chance for long-term survival? Should age play a factor so that a higher value is placed on a young person's life than on an older person's life? Should people whose lifestyles have caused their disease be just as likely to receive a transplant as someone else—say an alcoholic versus a nonalcoholic in the case of liver transplantation? Should a person who has already received a transplant be placed high on the list to receive another one if the first transplant fails? Given that organs are "donated," who owns the organs and who should decide on how they are allocated? Should patients from foreign countries be given an organ donated in the United States?

This chapter focuses on several questions surrounding organ allocation. Although the concepts of justice and fairness are priorities in considering the distribution of organs, not everyone agrees on exactly what is fair and just.

DISTRIBUTIVE JUSTICE

Because the lack of donor organs has ultimately led to many deaths, the issue of distributive justice is integral to organ allocation. The idea behind distributive justice is to allocate various goods in limited supply relative to demand and to ensure that everyone receives their fair share. Although the principles of distributive justice are complex and many-sided depending on the type of "goods" being considered, the theory does not endorse a single "right" way to distribute goods, especially in the case of lifesaving transplant organs. In reality, there are a number of ways that justification could be made for giving an organ to one particular individual over someone else. For example, organs could be allocated to each person as an equal share or according to criteria such as the individual's need, effort, contribution, or merit.

In the United States, the primary criteria established for receiving an organ is medical need, or the sickest patients first, followed closely by the probable long-term success of a transplant. This type of distributive justice criteria is sometimes referred to as striving for the "maximum benefit." On the surface, this approach to organ allocation appears to be fair because it tries to meet the immediate need of the sickest patients and also focuses on those who are most likely to benefit from the transplant. By taking into account these two vital factors, the goal is to avoid "wasting" organs.

The "sickest first" policy is relatively straightforward in that these patients are the most likely to die in a relatively short amount of time if they do not receive an organ. However, some argue that allocating such a scarce resource to those patients who are most ill is actually wasteful.

These patients, they argue, are less likely to survive and do well in the long term than a healthier patient who may be at the earlier stages of an illness. By factoring in the likelihood of long-term success, the organ-allocation process seeks to mitigate this argument.

Despite the apparent wisdom behind the maximum-benefit approach to distributive justice, some argue that the term "success" is difficult to define in terms of a lifesaving operation that requires such a scarce resource. For example, should success be based on how long the patient lives after receiving an organ or on how long the transplanted organ itself survives before the patient needs another transplant? If success is based on the number of years lived after a transplant, then the choice appears obvious when there are two equally sick patients who need a heart but who may be forty years apart in age. In a philosophical sense, the younger patient is "needier" because he or she has yet to live a life equally as full as the older patient. Furthermore, the younger patient has a higher chance of having more years of life gained overall than the older patient. On the other hand, this approach devalues the life of the older person. Critics argue that, regardless of age, the older patient's life has equal value to anyone else's and perhaps more value to some and society as a whole. For example, perhaps the older individual is an accomplished physician or scientific researcher. Although the younger person has the potential to accomplish great things for society, there is no guarantee that this will be the case.

Another issue in the definition of "success" could also be quality of life. Should a patient who has a chance for a higher quality of life than another patient receive priority? Of course, judgments about quality of life can be subjective and often stem from an individual's perspective of self-worth and ability to deal with difficulties in life. Many stories abound of people living with extremely debilitating diseases but who go on to achieve great personal satisfaction and also benefit others. In the end, because of the subjective nature of "success" beyond the idea of life and death, some people argue that basing organ distribution solely on maximum benefit is an opportunity for a number of unfair practices to come into play, including bias, favoritism, and even lying.

DOES EVERYONE *DESERVE* A TRANSPLANT?

One aspect that can be factored into a distributive justice system is the idea of equal access for all versus merit. Some would argue that certain segments of the population are more "deserving" of a transplant than others. For example, should someone who has led a relatively healthy life be on equal footing in the organ-allocation process with someone whose alcoholism caused the need for a new liver or whose smoking necessitated a new heart or lungs or both? Others would argue that if a person has reformed and no longer drinks or smokes, then we should not hold their past against them. However, opponents contend that these people are "bad investments" for the use of a limited resource. Because of their past abuse, the argument goes, they are more likely than other recipients to once again abuse alcohol or smoke cigarettes and, thus, damage their new organs. Such an issue arose in England in 2003 when famous English footballer and known alcoholic George Best received a liver transplant only to start drinking again within a year. Best died a relatively short time afterward.

Although it may seem a "common sense" approach to deny such people transplants, many physicians and ethicists do not agree. For a start, the estimation of "social worthiness" is not a factor that physicians think is ethical to employ in the treatment of patients, regardless of their illness or the amount of resources available. Furthermore, many would point out that both genetic and environmental factors are known to influence a person's likelihood of becoming an alcoholic and that it is unfair to discriminate against someone who has been "unlucky" in these aspects. In addition, there is no scientific data showing that alcoholics are more likely to drink after receiving a transplant than nonalcoholics. Opponents to such a worthiness approach also contend that programs for allocating organs employ a rigorous screening approach that, in the case of alcoholics, determines whether or not there is a good chance that the patient will stay clean and sober following their surgery and not suffer recidivism. They fear that taking into consideration individual worthiness opens a Pandora's box of problems, beginning with deciding who will ultimately make the decision of who is worthy and who is not.

Nevertheless, others argue that individual worthiness is a viable factor to consider because people who are clearly "worthy" individuals are biased against under the current system. For example, a person whose lifestyle has led to their need for an organ could have likely prevented their illness by choosing a healthier lifestyle. Furthermore, because of the illness that they have brought upon themselves, they are actually increasing the need for organs and depriving others of the chance to obtain one. Finally, proponents of considering "worthiness" in organ allocation point to studies that show that even though a return to drinking has not been proven to negatively affect the transplant, there is nevertheless a decreased chance of survival. Their belief is that an alcoholic or other type of addict is still much more likely to abuse substances than someone who has led a "clean and sober" life. For example, according to various studies, the rate of relapse in alcoholics who receive transplants ranges from 20 to 33 percent.

Prisoners and Transplantation

When it comes to the question of who is deserving to receive a scarce lifesaving resource, such as a transplanted organ, based on some estimation of "social worth," many would argue that giving a transplant to a prisoner is not ethical. A 2002 case in which a prison inmate in California became the first prisoner to receive a heart transplant sparked a debate over the use of the scarce commodity. Those against giving transplants to prisoners point out that the prison population in the United States is aging, which is increasing this population's need for health care services such as transplantation. Despite the fact that the U.S. Supreme Court ruled in the 1970s that prisoners were entitled to receive adequate medical care, many argue that giving them a rare transplanted organ goes above and beyond "adequate" care and deprives a law-abiding citizen of the chance for a lifesaving organ. They believe that prisoners forfeit all kinds of rights, such as the right to freedom, and should not gain new rights that others may be denied.

Those who argue that prisoners should have the right to a transplant point out that the idea of social worth is problematic, especially in the case of denying prisoners transplants, which forces transplant professionals to be an extension of the judicial system. For example, refusing a transplant to a prisoner can be equated with a type of death sentence. Furthermore, they point out that denying prisoners transplants means that those who run the allocation system must have some oversight of the system to ensure that it is conducted fairly in the case of these patients. Another factor to consider is the cost. Some argue that it is unfair to pay for a prisoner's transplant, which in the California case is estimated to ultimately cost the state over $1 million dollars, while law-abiding citizens who can't afford a transplant face almost certain death. (See the following section, "The Green Screen.")

THE GREEN SCREEN

For some, one of the most troubling aspects of the organ-allocation issue is the money factor. A 1993 Gallup Poll found that 58 percent of the respondents disagreed with a statement that a poor person in the same medical condition as a rich person has just as good of a chance of getting an organ transplant. Some subsequent high-profile cases have reinforced this public opinion. For example, baseball legend Mickey Mantle and former Pennsylvania governor Robert P. Casey rapidly received transplants shortly after being placed on a transplant waiting list. Although no evidence was uncovered to suggest that either of these people received preferential treatment, theirs and other similar cases raised red flags that preferential treatment was being given to certain patients, including those who are wealthy.

In fact, the ability to pay has a significant impact on more than those who are poor, without health insurance, or both. "It also can be an insuperable barrier to those with normally adequate health insurance, who still may have to pay many thousands of dollars in out-of-pocket expenses. As is attested by frequent stories in local and national media, when patients or their families cannot meet the costs of a transplant, beginning with an initial 'down payment,' . . . they often resort to desperate fund-raising efforts" (Fox and Swazey, 1992).

Like almost all types of health care in the United States, money does play a role in access to organ transplant waiting lists. In fact, a patient usually has to demonstrate the ability to pay transplant-associated costs to gain access to a list. The reality is that patients who are unable to pay for a transplant either out of their own pocket or through insurances can be denied the transplant when hospitals cannot afford to pay for the surgery and long-term recovery of the patient.

In the realm of organ transplantation, the ability to pay raises some unique ethical issues. The 1986 federal Task Force on Organ Transplantation argued for eliminating the ability to pay as a criterion for receiving a transplant because of the unique aspect of organ transplantation that relies on public donations. The task force believed that "it is unfair, even exploitative to ask rich and poor alike to donate organs if only the rich have any effective chance of receiving organ transplants in cases of medical need" (Childress, 1996).

In fact, according to a 2006 article in the *Journal of the American College of Cardiology* titled "Health Insurance and Cardiac Transplantation: A Call for Reform," an estimated 25 percent of donated organs come from the uninsured, leading to the following question: is it fair to ask someone to donate an organ if that same person does not have a realistic chance of receiving one if he or she needs it? Many argue that because organ transplants are "gifts of life" based on public altruism to make organs available, a public policy that asks everyone to donate but gives organs only to those who can pay is indefensible.

Others, however, note that unequal access to health care is a fact of life in the United States. They also point out that not all transplant centers turn away uninsured patients and that many can help them pay for the treatment and follow-up care or at least try to arrange some kind of help in finding a way to fund their treatment. Nevertheless, others contend that individual transplant centers often conduct a close scrutiny of a patient's finances. In addition, wealthy patients also have the ability to investigate different centers to get higher on a transplant waiting list or to get placed on several lists at different centers while poorer patients must go to the closest center and are bound by the policies within that center. Finally, some would argue that it is truly wasteful to offer transplants to people who can't afford to pay for the transplant or the follow-up drug regimen and care. They contend that organs allocated to these people will ultimately be wasted because the patients are not able to afford to pay for the drugs needed to keep him alive.

SHOULD DONORS GET PRIORITY?

The primary problem surrounding donor-organ shortages is not that people are failing to die under the circumstances that allow their organs to be harvested. Rather, too few people have agreed to have their organs donated. Although efforts have been made to increase the percentage of the population that agrees to donate, the numbers remain far short of need. As a result, some propose that priority for access to donated organs should be given to people who have agreed themselves to donate their own organs upon their deaths.

The argument basically states that altruism in organ donation has failed and that the organ-allocation system will benefit from not only giving priority to people who have agreed to be organ donors but also perhaps even denying organs to anyone who has not agreed to donate their own organs upon death. Proponents of this approach believe that under the current system people do not perceive a benefit to themselves for becoming a cadaveric donor. Changing the allocation system to give priority to potential organ donors, they argue, would be an incentive for more people to donate and, thus, save thousands of lives.

Proponents of a new allocation system that considers organ-donor status believe it is simply a matter of "justice," contending that an ethically relevant difference exists between those who do donate and those who do not. For example, they cite a similar example in which the United Network for Organ Sharing (UNOS) gives people who have been living donors additional points to move them up on the waiting list should they need a transplant. It is only fair, they contend, that people who agree to be organ donors upon their death receive at the very least similar treatment. They add that new programs like LifeSharers, which allows members to allocate their organs to other members in case one of them should die, are already in place.

An example of a program employing a similar philosophy in organ allocation already exists in several countries and in Europe, where in the 1990s members of the European Community, now known as the European Union, collaborated in an organ-sharing network but dropped countries with low donation rates from the network. Finally, such a policy, proponents point out, could be implemented without initial legislative action. In a 1993 white paper titled "Preferred Status for Organ Donors," a UNOS Ethics Committee concluded, "A trial could be implemented without requiring any alteration in existing legislation" (Burdick, 1993).

Opponents to changing organ-allocation policies in this direction believe that the approach fosters "selfishness" in what has long been considered an altruistic act. Furthermore, they believe that selfishness alone is not enough to make current nondonors register to be donors. They note that the chances of a "reward" are actually minimal given that the far majority of people do not need transplants. Religious and esthetic reasons also account for why some people do not sign up to be organ donors, and a reward system will not change their outlook, say opponents.

Another argument used against giving priority to "future" potential organ donors is that "the evidence that might support ruling someone out of organ eligibility is not available when the transplant decision has to be made. Intentions are easy to conceal, and anyone who signs a donor card now can tear it up later" (Kuhse and Singer, 1998). As a result, placing sanctions on those who have not agreed to donate could be highly unfair.

The UNOS Ethics Committee white paper also pointed out other potential disadvantages to the system. For example, the committee commented that a public perception that the preference to potential donors is too great might lead them to consider the system to be unfair and easily manipulated. Furthermore, if not enough advantage is given to donors, they could see the offer as having no real meaning or being an insincere tactic designed to gain higher donation rates. The committee also delineated a scenario that raises further ethical questions:

> Consider the scenario of two medically similar patients, for whom preferred status would be the tie-breaker. One patient has signed an organ donor card, but has had a life of doing harm to society, robbing and beating others. The other patient has lived an exemplary life, has contributed financially and personally to medical causes including transplantation, and therefore has directly benefited many other people, but has not felt comfortable with agreeing to organ donation. Is there justice in the former person receiving the organ, allowing the one arbitrary fact of opting into the system to override all the other comparative points, which would tend the choice toward the latter? (Burdick, 1993)

Foreign Transplant Recipients

At a meeting on March 2, 2006, the Organ Procurement Transplant Network (OPTN) and the United Network for Organ Sharing (UNOS) declared St. Vincent Medical Center in Los Angeles to be a "Member Not in Good Standing." The sanction was imposed because of the discovery that hospital surgeons had bypassed nine eligible patients higher on its waiting list to improperly arrange a liver transplant for a Saudi national who was not among the neediest patients and whose government paid $339,000 for the operation and follow-up care.

Some critics of the organ transplantation system in the United States believe that it is unfair to give such a rare resource as donor organs to foreign patients. Furthermore, citing such examples as the St. Vincent case, they believe that rich foreigners, who may pay as much as ten times the price that local patients pay for the same operation, often "buy" their way to the top of transplant waiting lists. However, hospital officials do have the discretion to put foreign citizens, including illegal immigrants, on the national waiting list for a transplant. Currently, UNOS policy allows for up to 5 percent of organ recipients to be patients from other countries.

Those in favor of allowing foreigners to receive some transplants believe that it is fair to give some organs to these patients because they also donate organs to U.S. patients. They also point out that, as a percentage, U.S. citizens donate fewer organs than they receive each year. For example, in 2001, 96.2 percent of the transplant recipients in the United States were U.S. citizens, but only 94.8 percent of the organ donors were citizens as opposed to permanent residents, non-resident foreigners, and others. Furthermore, some argue that denying transplants to foreign nationals would unfairly discriminate against and punish patients from poorer countries that cannot afford to run their own transplantation programs. Finally, they believe that allowing some foreign nationals to receive transplants in the United States is a sign of goodwill and a common bond among members of the worldwide community.

In the end, perceived and real imperfections in organ-allocation policies can be directly traced to the lack of donor organs. Most likely, until there are enough organs for everyone, biases and politics will continue to influence rankings within the system to some degree. Similarly, the federal government, the public, and medical professionals will continue to make organ allocation one of the most intensely scrutinized aspects of modern medicine. Because organ transplantation rests on a foundation of altruism and trust, it is essential that such analyses continue.

CHAPTER 7

Xenotransplantation: Animal Use and Infectious Disease

In 1997 surgeons drilled an approximately quarter-inch hole into the skull of Parkinson's disease patient Jim Finn, inserted a six-inch needle, and then injected twelve million fetal pig cells into his brain. They hoped that the cells would "take" and reinitiate the lost brain functions associated with Finn's neurological disease. Within six months, Finn—whose Parkinson's had reached the stage at which he could no longer walk, talk, or use his hands— was walking independently and able to stand and sit in a chair. He also went on to regain his ability to talk. However, no one has been able to definitively declare that the transplant initiated Finn's partial recovery, and other patients in the same clinical trial received no or little benefits from the procedure. Nevertheless, in 2003, six years after the operation, Finn called the procedure "a miracle for me" during an interview on the Public Broadcasting System's (PBS) online companion to *Religion and Ethics Newsweekly*, one of PBS's television programs. Finn also noted, "When you are faced with dying, you would be amazed as to what you would agree to" (PBS, 2003).

Xenotransplantation, or transplantation across species, is seen as a potential answer to the problem of donor shortages. Although some research focuses on tissues and cells, scientists and surgeons are also investigating the use of whole organs from other species for transplantation. Initial efforts in whole-organ xenotransplantation included six chimpanzee kidneys transplanted into humans in the early 1960s, a baboon heart transplanted into the infant "Baby Fae" in 1984 (see sidebar), and baboon livers transplanted into two patients in 1992. Although all of these efforts failed, scientists noted that most of the patients died of infections related to their immunosuppression and not directly to organ malfunctioning.

Baby Fae and Informed Consent

On October 26, 1984, Baby Fae was born prematurely with an underdeveloped left side of the heart, known as hypoplastic left-heart syndrome, which is normally fatal within a short time after birth. Surgeon Leonard L. Bailey and colleagues at the Loma Linda University Medical Center in California tried to save Baby Fae by transplanting a donor baboon's heart into her twelve days after birth. Bailey and others were hoping that the "immature" condition of the baby's immune system would allow Baby Fae to accept the transplanted organ.

The new heart initially worked well, beating on its own and changing Baby Fae from a sickly-looking infant into a healthy baby with a pinkish glow. Baby Fae made headlines around the world but died on November 15, 1984, from heart and kidney failure resulting from an immunological response.

The Baby Fae case early on highlighted several controversies surrounding xenotransplantation, and one of the biggest focused on the idea of informed consent. Informed consent is a legal condition in which an individual is giving consent based on an understanding of the facts and implications of his or her actions. In the medical arena, informed consent requires that significant risks of a procedure be disclosed, as well as risks that would be of particular importance to that patient.

Questions were raised about the quality and extent of information provided to Baby Fae's parents for their informed consent. Most notably, some observers believed the parents were not fully or correctly informed about the benefits of a surgical repair procedure available to repair left hypoplastic hearts. Called the Norwood procedure, it had been developed in 1979 by William Norwood at Children's Hospital in Boston. Critics of the xenotransplant argued that the data available on xenotransplantations at the time of Baby Fae's operation indicated that the likelihood of success was extremely low and that the Norwood procedure represented a better chance for survival. Another concern about the informed-consent process was "the instability apparent in the parents' financial situation and personal lives which could have increased their vulnerability to manipulation or coercion" (Mistichelli, 1985). The controversy led a National Institutes of Health (NIH) committee to review the procedures involved in informed consent in the Baby Fae case, and the review found weaknesses in the procedure, including overstating the baby's chances for long-term survival.

Bailey and others have countered that the Baby Fae case was handled ethically. They also note that, in their opinion, Baby Fae did not die in vain but helped launch successful infant heart allo-transplantation, which has achieved an approximately 80 percent success rate.

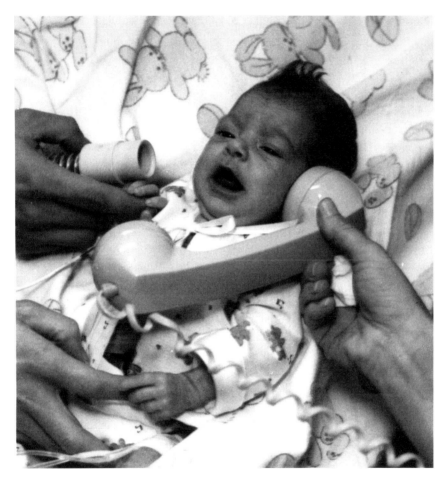

Xenotransplant recipient Baby Fae listens to her mother's voice over the phone just 13 days after the infant's historic heart transplant. (AP Images)

More recently, scientists have turned to pigs as a potential source of human organs and therapeutic cells for transplantation. Using pigs avoids the ethical issues associated with killing primates, which are closely related biologically to humans, are considered intelligent, and include some endangered species. (Nonhuman primates are still used, however, in transplantation and other medical research.) Pigs also reproduce at a much faster rate than primates, are easier to care for, and are less likely to transmit viruses to humans that could turn into a pandemic. For example, the origins of the human immunodeficiency virus (HIV) and acquired immune deficiency syndrome (AIDS) involved transmission of a virus that lived harmlessly in our primate biological cousins but turned deadly after gaining entrance into human hosts.

Nevertheless, several important controversies surround xenotransplantation. Some question the right to use animals as replacement parts. Others are concerned about our human identity coupled with spiritual and cultural values. Finally, the most daunting issue may be the potential to accidentally let loose or create a deadly virus that turns into a pandemic. Because nonhuman primates have been deemed largely unsuitable as organ donors, this chapter focuses primarily on the issues surrounding the research involving pig organs.

SHOULD WE HARVEST ORGANS FROM ANIMALS?

On the surface, the argument against using animals as sources of transplant organs is negated by the fact that a large portion of the human population eats animals not just for survival but also for enjoyment. Most religions have agreed that the use of animals for the "good of man" is appropriate and morally sanctioned. Even Islam and Judaism, both of which forbid eating pork, approve of xenotransplantation as long as the animals are treated humanely. Religions that take a negative view of transplantation, such as Buddhism and Hinduism, still leave the choice up to the individual.

Nevertheless, many people and groups still claim a moral ground when they question the use of animals as "spare parts" for humans. Animal rights activists would argue that "two wrongs do not make a right," noting that our husbandry of animals for food dates back thousands of years and is an engrained part of our societies and habits. They point out that current research animals are already dying from failed experiments and, they believe, suffering a number of traumas in the process, including major surgery, internal hemorrhages, isolation in small cages, infections, and vomiting and diarrhea because of the use of immunosuppressant drugs. In 2000 leaked internal documents from a medical research company in Great Britain revealed that the company Imutran financed over a period of several years research experiments in xenotransplantation that ultimately destroyed 420 monkeys and nearly 50 baboons. On average, the baboons, who had pig hearts implanted either in their neck or abdomen, survived slightly less than two weeks. Although the debate continues as to how much these animals suffered, those opposed to xenotransplantation say that any infliction of pain, suffering, and death is unacceptable.

At the basis of the argument against using animals is the idea of their consciousness. Nonhuman primates, for example, are considered to have a high level of consciousness and, although not on par with humans, similar psychosocial traits as humans, including a greater capacity for suffering than other animals because of their level of self-awareness. Other animals, however, are also thought to be relatively intelligent, such as our pet cats and dogs. Does this consideration apply to pigs? Over the years various stories have appeared in newspapers and on television about people with pet pigs, sometimes delighting or disgusting viewers with the sight of a 300-pound pig lounging on the sofa. Animal rights activists point out that pigs, to a degree, are intelligent and sensitive animals that may be equated as being on the same intellectual level as dogs. If dogs were being used in this manner, they argue, the outcry would be deafening.

Scientists and xenotransplantation proponents say they understand the concerns but stress that animal research is the very basis of modern medical advances. For example, almost all drugs licensed for use have been tested for toxicity in animals, including vaccines that fought off the deadly smallpox and debilitating poliomyelitis. Because we already use pigs as a food source, proponents believe that we are merely extending that use to mediate human pain and suffering. Finally, they point out that tissues derived from the pig heart have been used for three decades in heart valve operations.

Nevertheless, those opposed to xenotransplantation stress that the animals' quality of life is inadequately low because of how they are raised. In reality, the transplant organs do not come from pigs per se but rather six-month-old piglets. It as at this point in the pigs' growth that the organs are at optimal size for transplantation. Animal rights activists note that these animals are separated from their mothers by a type of cesarean section at a very young age and are raised in sterile and unnatural conditions with a low quality of life until they are killed. Scientists argue, however, that the pigs live perfectly healthy lives and are well looked after. In terms of product, they say they want quality organs and that such organs come from happy and healthy animals.

A Question of Identity?

Although asking "Who am I?" may seem like an existential question, some do question whether transplanting animal organs into humans is tampering with an individual's personal identity, as well as society's view of what it means to be human. On the one hand, transplanting pig cells might have little effect on personal identity, but receiving an animal's heart or eyes could have a significantly different psychological impact. Is there a point at which the transplant recipient would feel less human in some way?

Xenotransplantation could also affect our societal paradigm, that is, our collective values, attitudes, beliefs, myths, and symbols. Will it cause us to have a different and perhaps lesser view of both our individual and collective lives? For example, ethicists note that we have an "integrated" theory of personal identity that helps us see ourselves as unique human beings. Efforts such as xenotransplantation could move us toward a "modular" approach to personal identity, in which we perceive ourselves more simply as a collection of interchangeable parts. However, some ethicists note that xenotransplantation could also increase our sense of awe and wonder about ourselves and all life.

Opponents believe that much of the interest in xenotransplantation is economically based and driven by those seeking to make a profit. They believe that there are numerous alternatives to xenotransplantation, including expanding the human donor pool through better education efforts and establishing extensive laws such as universal consent to take an organ from a deceased individual unless otherwise notified. Indeed, much of the effort in developing animals for transplantation resides in the private sector or in private-academic partnerships that could be extremely lucrative, making millions and perhaps billions of dollars within the industry as a whole. Proponents counter, however, that many companies make large profits in the health care industry and that the bottom line is saving lives.

OPENING PANDORA'S BOX?

Moral arguments alone are probably insufficient to prevent xenotransplantation. The animal rights movement dates back to the late nineteenth and early twentieth centuries when anti-vivisectionists protested surgery on animals for physiological and pathological research. Nevertheless, medical research involving animals has continued. Because most religions and societies have condoned animal use for human betterment and animals are slaughtered every day for food, saving human lives is still likely to trump concerns for animals in a large majority of the human population.

In addition to moral arguments against transplantation, however, is a practical concern regarding a potentially disastrous outcome that involves risk not only to transplant patients but also to the public at large. Zoonosis is the transmission of infectious agents from one species to another and is sometimes referred to as xenozoonoses in the case of xenotransplantation. Cross-species infections are usually caused by viruses, bacteria, and prions (a protein particle similar to a virus but without nucleic acid) transferring from animal to animal and then to humans. For example, the HIV that leads to AIDS is a retrovirus and a human version of the simian immunodeficiency virus (SIV) found in infected chimpanzees. The transference of infectious viruses and bacteria also occurs in human-to-human transplantation.

The transplant community's eventual decision to largely forego the use of nonhuman primate organs for the present is avoiding a significant concern. Nonhuman primates harbor both known and potentially unknown viruses that might readily adapt to the human body and spread throughout the population in a manner similar to HIV, that is, in the form of a previously unknown disease or a new form of a disease. On the other hand, people have been in contact with pigs for centuries with little evidence of disease transference, although pigs can contract influenza from humans. In 1997, however, researchers showed that the porcine endogenous retrovirus (or PERV), which resides in most pigs, can infect human cells in the laboratory setting. In 2000 another study revealed that PERV was transmitted during the transplantation of pancreatic pig cells into immunosuppressed diabetic mice.

A primary concern is that PERV is a retrovirus that has the ability to mutate and recombine easily within a cell. Ultimately, any infections or their symptoms might not show up for a considerable time, perhaps even decades if patients live that long. In addition, pig cells and organs that are transplanted into humans may contain not only PERV but also infectious agents that are currently unknown. Already, scientists have found more than sixty porcine infectious agents with a potential to cause disease in humans. A 2004 finding at the Mayo Clinic in Minnesota also showed that human and animal DNA can fuse together and form hybrids, further raising concerns about the unknown potential to create new and deadly diseases. To date, primary medical concerns surround the potential for an infection to produce an AIDS-like virus or cancers such as lymphomas and leukemias.

Some opponents to xenotransplantation say that the potential risk of spreading infectious diseases into a general population is too much of a public health danger to proceed, considering that thousands or perhaps millions of people could die. For most viruses of known concern, researchers and xenotransplant organ developers have developed careful control measures to prevent infectious agents from developing and being passed on to the human recipients. These measures include a sterile environment and routine monitoring of the pigs and those who handle them. Scientists have also developed recent methods to detect these viruses and infections, but many still cannot be identified and constitute a potentially serious unknown risk.

Opponents also argue that transplantation presents the ideal environment for introducing viruses because many natural barriers are blocked by the immunosuppressive regimen that transplant recipients receive. The genetic manipulation of pigs to make them more "acceptable" to human immune systems might also increase the risk of virus transmission according to some experts. For example, some of the human genes being bred into transgenic pigs can code for proteins to act as virus receptors.

Transplant professionals contend that the likelihood of viral or bacterial infections occurring in pigs raised in an extremely controlled "pathogen-free" environment is exceptionally low. They also note that none of the 200 or so human patients who have received experimental pig-cell transplant therapies have been infected with any infectious agents, including PERV. Furthermore, patients are monitored closely. For example, before Parkinson's disease patient Jim Finn could receive the experimental injection of porcine fetal cells, he had to agree to undergo lifelong blood monitoring and not to engage in unprotected sex or father children.

On the other side of the argument, opponents point out that, as an endogenous retrovirus, PERV resides in the DNA of the pig chromosomes and remains there no matter how clean the pigs are kept. Furthermore, monitoring programs can be ineffective, especially when dealing with huge populations. For example, monitoring HIV patients does not prevent people from having unprotected sex even though they know that it is the primary way to transmit the virus. If transplanting pig organs becomes successful, critics of the practice believe that the number of patients would be far too great for monitoring to ensure adherence to strict guidelines that are designed both to protect the patients and to prevent the transmission of diseases to others. They also note the potential development of "xenotourism" as hindering monitoring capabilities. On the other hand,

Playing God: Transgenic Animals and Xenotransplantation
Current models of xenotransplantation are based on genetically altered, or transgenic, animals. For example, pigs are being bred with human genes designed to make the animals' organs and tissues more acceptable to the human immune system. With modern advances in the ability to manipulate the genes that hold the codes for cell differentiation and functioning, some have expressed concerns over tampering with the natural order of the world. For example, there is concern that the process could negatively impact the environment and a wide range of animals through interbreeding. On the other hand, some argue that the scenario is highly unlikely because of the well-regulated, relatively small-scale operations that would be needed to breed animals for xenotransplantation. They also note that a single gene does not contain the essence of any human or animal and that species change with evolution.

some believe that having a well-regulated xenotransplantation program would reduce the risk of xenotourism to less well-regulated countries, where transplanted organs may contain infectious diseases that could be brought back to the patient's home country.

Another point made by opponents to xenotransplantation is that even if the risk is "small" as judged by transplant and infectious disease professionals, the potential harm could be significant in terms of dealing with thousands of people infected with viruses. The potential for disaster is real, opponents contend, referring to the influenza pandemic of 1918, which seemed to kill the young and healthy as well as the old and sickly. Most estimates are that the pandemic killed somewhere between twenty and forty million people worldwide. Although modern medical science has much more in its armament to fend off such catastrophes, technological advances that can transport people, and therefore viruses, around the world in a matter of hours could counteract modern medical science. For example, the spread of AIDS has killed approximately one-half million people in the United States and approximately fourteen million worldwide.

IS IT A RISK WORTH TAKING?

Life is full of apparent risks that each of us takes often, if not every day. Driving a car is a risk; so is skiing. The goal is not to live in a risk-free world, which is impossible. Rather, point out ethicists, the goal is to develop as much control as possible over the risks taken. To date, the transplant community has shown restraint in its xenotransplantation efforts, such as when Thomas E. Starzl at the University of Pittsburgh Medical Center halted baboon-to-human kidney transplant procedures in 1992 because of immunosuppression and organ rejection issues.

Scientists currently acknowledge that it is not possible to completely eradicate the risk of PERV transmission to humans, as well as other potential infectious invaders. Nevertheless, because of its therapeutic potential, xenotransplantation is likely to move forward. As a result, more attention is being paid to governmental controls over xenotransplantation experiments and, if successful, clinical use. In the United States, for example, the Centers for Disease Control and Prevention and the National Institutes of Health have issued guidelines for research in xenotransplantation, including regulations on proper product sources and on animal screening and qualifications. In addition, most Western nations have laws that outline humane and safe treatment of animals in research environments, but there are contentions over whether these laws are adequate and should be improved to benefit the animals.

Before clinical trials begin on a widespread basis, scientists must make considerable strides in their research. Ethicists note that they also must carefully evaluate whether clinical use is justified by a measurable amount of success. What constitutes "success" is debatable. So far, researchers have demonstrated graft survival times in animal models of xenotransplantation that are comparable to allotransplantation (between the same species) prior to 1967. For example, current survival in these models is from a few weeks to three months. Many experts would like to see at least "routine" survival rates of ninety days before moving on to clinical trials with humans, keeping in mind that research patients involved in experimental therapies such as xenotransplantation are likely to already be in a life-and-death situation.

Those who believe xenotransplantation is a serious health risk to the general population warn that once the genie is out of the bottle, it may difficult to contain widespread infections of some unknown or mutated virus. Others contend that xenotransplantation is one of the best hopes for acquiring enough organs to save countless lives and that the benefits far outweigh the risks, which they perceive as minimal. Because thousands of people die each year without receiving a lifesaving organ, scientists will continue to explore the potential of xenotransplantation. The ethical debates surrounding animal care and the potential spread of infectious diseases will also continue, serving to heighten awareness about research involving animals and the need for stringent safety measures.

CHAPTER 8

Living Donors: Giving until It Hurts?

Danny Boone and Michael Hurewitz did not think that they would be making the ultimate sacrifice when they decided to become living donors. Each man donated part of his liver to save the life of another and expected to fully recover. Their expectations were based on the fact that the liver is unique among organs in that a partial liver will regenerate to its normal size and functioning in about two weeks. Nevertheless, each man died as a result of his decision. Boone, it turns out, had several hidden medical problems that should have precluded him from being a liver donor, including fatty liver disease, an enlarged liver and spleen, and celiac stenosis (constriction of blood flow to the liver by a ligament). Despite five more surgeries in an attempt to save his life, Boone died three weeks after entering the hospital in 1999.

Michael Hurewitz, on the other hand, was in good health. Nevertheless, he died in 2002 only three days after donating a portion of his liver to his brother Adam, who went on to recover fully. Hurewitz's death has largely been attributed to poor postoperative care by inexperienced residents working on a transplant unit that housed thirty-four patients at the time. Following her husband's death, Vickie Hurewitz became a vocal activist proposing that a moratorium be placed on living donor transplants.

One of the primary tenets of medical practice has been *primun non nocere*, that is, "do no harm." In the case of Boone and Hurewitz and thousands of other living donors, this "golden rule" of medicine is being tested because no physically tangible benefit exists for an individual who undergoes the risks of surgery as a living donor. Although the risk of dying as a living donor of a liver is approximately 1 percent, many consider this rate unacceptable. It is also important to note that, in addition to the mortality rate, the morbidity rate (that is, the rate of having a medical problem or an unhealthy side effect) is estimated to be about 30 percent. Unlike living donors for livers, the mortality risk is much lower for living kidney donors, at about one in 2,500 to one in 4,000. Nevertheless, the risk still exists as evidenced by the fact that some kidney donors have died as a result of perioperative (at or around the time of surgery) complications, and at least one has ended up in a persistent vegetative state.

Although each individual generally has full autonomy over his or her own body, the issue of living donor transplantation raises a complex set of moral problems. Even though many agree that living donors have some right to take a certain amount of risk, questions arise over whether people truly do understand the risks of being a living donor and the long-term impact it may have on their health, longevity, comfort, and overall quality of life. Other questions include the following: Is or can coercion be involved in a person's decision to donate, especially to a relative? Does advertising for live donors from strangers cross ethical boundaries and perhaps even lead to a "waste" of organs? Can living donors not related to the organ recipient by family or social ties stipulate that their organs only be given to people of a certain race, religion, or ethnic background? Are enough societal and institutional safeguards in place to truly protect living donors?

Although most transplant physicians and those in the ethical community agree that the preferred route of organ donation is to obtain organs from people who have agreed to donate after their death, once again the specter of low organ-donation rates looms. As a result, more and more transplant centers are turning to live donors to help solve the shortage problem.

A BRIEF HISTORY OF LIVING DONATION

The very foundation of transplantation rests on living donation. In 1954 Ronald Herrick donated part of his kidney for transplantation into his twin brother Richard to help treat Richard's fatal kidney disease, marking the first successful human transplant case (see Chapter 1). For many years, "living-related kidney transplants" were performed primarily between living donors and recipients who were usually related by blood. The ability to match donor organs with recipients is largely based on histocompatibility, or human leukocyte antigen (HLA) compatibility, which is the degree of similarity between some antigens that plays a large role in determining the likelihood of a transplant or blood transfusion succeeding. Because HLA compatibility also can exist between unrelated individuals, nonrelated living kidney donors began to be used more in the 1970s as transplantation progressed and the transplant community broadened its search for suitable donor organs. Eventually, the improvement of immuno-suppressive drugs led to an even broader range of compatibility between people so that today more people than ever have the potential to be living donors for transplant patients.

According to the United Network for Organ Sharing (UNOS), approxi-mately 50 percent of all U.S. donor kidneys in the twenty-first century have come from living donors. The operation is relatively simple, and the donor's remaining kidney can compensate for the missing kidney and do the work once performed by two kidneys. As a result, the procedure is considered relatively safe, considering that all invasive surgeries contain a certain amount of risk, such as infections and other complications.

Living donors were first used for liver transplantation in the late 1980s as part of an effort to treat children, and the process usually involved transplanting part of the parent's liver to the child. These pediatric trans-plants involved transplantation of the liver's left lobe. Subsequent advances in surgical techniques led to adult-to-adult liver transplantations involving the right lobe. However, the adult procedure is much more tech-nically difficult than the pediatric surgery, largely because it removes a larger segment of the liver. As a result, adult donors for adult recipients face a higher risk of complications than do the donors in living donor transplants targeting children. In 2004 living organ donors provided a lobe of the liver for approximately 320 transplants in the United States.

In addition to transplants of the kidney and liver, fifteen living donor transplants involving a lobe of the lung were performed in 2004. Experts generally agree that people can donate a portion of the lung and still main-tain complete functioning of their own lungs. Overall, of the 14,154 organ donors in the United States in 2004, 7,150 were deceased organ donors, and 7,004 were living organ donors, an increase of 2.4 percent over 2003. Nevertheless, this increase was smaller than in recent years, including the three previous years when living kidney donors outnumbered deceased donors. According to the Organ Procurement and Transplantation Network (OPTN), the other types of transplants that can be performed between liv-ing donors and recipients include the following:

- Pancreas: People can donate a part of the pancreas, which does not regenerate, but donors usually have little problem with reduced functioning.
- Intestine: It is possible to donate a portion of the intestine, but the operation is rarely performed at this time.

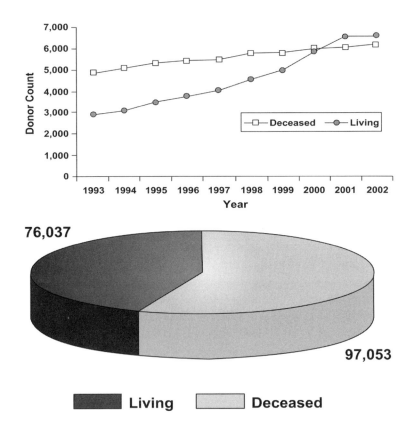

Figure 8.1

As the above graph illustrates, the total number of living donors was larger than the number of deceased donors for the first time 2001, with 6,560 living donors versus 6,081 deceased donors. The trend continued in 2002, during which there were 6,618 living donors versus 6,182 deceased donors. The Organ Procurement and Transplantation Network (OPTN) points out that it may be significant that the number of living donors changed minimally between 2001 and 2002 (6,560 versus 6,618) because it may indicate a trend that is in marked contrast with the preceding five years, during which the number of living donors increased annually by 500 to 1,000 donors. According to OPTN, this new trend may indicate a stabilization of the number of people deciding to become living donors. (Data gathered from the Organ Procurement and Transplantation Network Web site at http://www.optn.org, accessed June 14, 2006).

The pie chart is based on current OPTN data as reported on December 9, 2005, for the time period from January 1, 1988 to September 30, 2005. It illustrates the total number of living versus deceased donors during this time period. (Data gathered from the United Network for Organ Sharing Web site at http://www.unos.org, accessed June 14, 2006).

SAFETY, INFORMED CONSENT, AND THE RISK-BENEFIT RATIO

Although several ethical issues surround living donor transplantation, the primary concern remains donor safety. Few would disagree that the process of removing part of a person's organ is a major surgery that, regardless of the surgeon's skill, ultimately exposes the donor to potentially serious health problems, not to mention the immediate pain and recovery time that the donor experiences regardless of the operation's success. In the case of liver transplants, donors must also undergo invasive tests to ensure they are suitable donors, and these tests also have some associated risks. In effect, the donor bears all of the significant risks; the transplant recipient has nothing to lose because the donation is required to save his or her life.

What bothers many who question the validity of living donor transplants is the issue of informed consent. Informed consent is the process by which patients become fully informed so that they can make choices about their health care. The process stems from the recognized legal and ethical rights of patients to have control over their own bodies. However, can living donors really make a fully informed consent decision about donating? Critics point out that little information is available on the long-term outcome for living donors because the United States has not required the same record-keeping for living donor transplantation that is required for cadaveric organ donation. As a result, relatively little long-term follow-up data is available concerning the potential complications that a living donor might face.

Although UNOS requests that centers complete follow-up forms on living donors at six months and one year following surgery, this requirement still does not address long-term effects, and centers have reported that approximately 37 percent of living donors were lost to follow-up within one year of the transplant in comparison with only a 1 percent rate of lost follow-up for recipients. Critics suggest that the lack of concrete data concerning the effects on living donors compromises the entire informed consent procedure. Furthermore, some contend that potential living donors may have a difficult time figuring out the true meanings of potential risks when confronted by broad statistical data that they must apply to their own individual circumstances.

In the discussion of the ethics of living donor transplants, much of the argument surrounds the idea of the risk-benefit ratio. In other words, do the benefits outweigh the risks? For example, transplant recipients from living donors typically experience shorter waiting times, are assured of good graft quality, and also appear to have a better chance of survival both in the short-term and the long-term. Although many people see all the benefits of the operation going to the transplant recipient and all the risks being taken by

---

Kant and Organ Transplantation

Although the eighteenth-century philosopher Immanuel Kant died in 1804, long before organ transplantation became a reality, the respected thinker did weigh in on the subject of living donations, although he was referring primarily to the idea of tooth transplantation. According to Kant, individuals have the moral duty to preserve themselves according to their basic natures. For Kant, this represented the most fundamental argument against suicide other than an individual's religious beliefs. Kant also said that people had a moral obligation not to perform self-mutilation. Although Kant recognized the medical need to remove body parts and organs if they were injured or diseased, he believed that the donation of these parts by a living donor, whether for monetary gain or otherwise, was a form of self-mutilation and went against the imperative that people not use themselves simply as a means to an end. As a result, as part of his Principle of Humanity, Kant argued that any living person who donates a part of himself or herself is in essence committing "partial suicide." Though this view of Kantian-based bioethics is pervasive, some argue that live organ donation does not necessarily violate Kant's beliefs. They contend that organ donation is actually in some cases morally commendable based on Kant's concepts of active beneficence as mutual aid.

---

the donor, many others point out that the donor also receives some significant benefits from the procedure. People who agree to become living donors do undergo an intense physical, which is something of a benefit in terms of detecting any potential health problems the donor may have. According to proponents of living donation, however, the primary benefits are the psychological, emotional, and spiritual rewards, all of which lead to an increased sense of self-esteem. As a result, they point out, the ultimate risk-benefit ratio depends largely on the donors' personal value judgments. Ultimately, say proponents of the procedure, it is up to the prospective donor to decide whether the risk is worth it in order to achieve what they see as the ultimate good of saving someone's life.

FRIENDS, NEIGHBORS, COUNTRYMEN

Although living donations began primarily as donations made from a person to a terminally ill relative, the process eventually came to encompass nonrelated donors who felt a bond with the recipient in other ways, such as through personal friendship or through being part of a shared community, such as a church organization. These types of donations are called directed donations to a loved one or "friend." Because of the dire need for organs, this group of donors has further expanded to include nondirected donations, which involves a living donor giving an organ to a general organ pool for transplantation into the next recipient at the top of an organ donor waiting list.

Each type of donation raises some distinct ethical questions. Although relatives or "friends" of transplant recipients appear to be motivated only by altruistic concerns, some fear that relatives and friends who are reluctant to become donors may have their decisions unduly influenced by intense social pressures within the broader family context to donate. Although there is no universally recognized moral obligation for one family member to donate an organ to another in order to keep the ill family member alive, a sense of personal responsibility does exist for many. Most ethicists agree that this ethical dilemma applies primarily to family members and somewhat to friends rather than to living donors who are strangers. As a result, family members may feel compelled to donate without full consideration of what the long-term consequences for themselves might be. Of course, physicians and transplant centers do have the right to refuse live donors if they think the donors are being pressured in some way and really do not want to donate. It should also be noted that physicians have a moral obligation to reject live donors if they do not think the chance of success is significant.

Although living donors who participate in nondirected donations targeting the general organ candidate pool do not face the "obligation" pressures sometimes applied to family and friends, many note that it is important to carefully scrutinize the "radical altruism that motivates a person to make a potentially life-threatening sacrifice for a stranger" (Truog, 2005). For example, transplant centers must make sure that these donors are psychologically competent. Are psychological factors present to make them believe that they are somehow "obligated" to donate or perhaps must potentially "sacrifice" themselves for others in some way? Other issues that need to be considered are whether "the person [is] trying to compensate for depression or low self-esteem, seeking media attention, or harboring hopes of becoming involved in the life of the recipient" (Truog, 2005).

Although these are important considerations, proponents also point out that agreeing to become a living donor for a complete stranger may be the highest level of altruistic donation. The ultimate good that is achieved by saving someone's life, they contend, must be an important factor in the equation. As long as the individual undergoes comprehensive psychological testing and counseling, and anonymity is maintained between the donor and recipient, proponents argue that such donations are ethically justifiable based on the individual's right to autonomy over his or her own body.

DIRECTED LIVING DONATIONS: ENTERING THE GREY AREA

A relatively recent but rapidly growing area of living organ donation involves directed donations to strangers. Such donations must still be based on the notion of altruism and are not allowed by law to involve an exchange of money or other material benefit to the donor (see Chapter 5). Nevertheless, in addition to the ethical questions surrounding nondirected donations, this aspect of living donation raises a series of unique ethical dilemmas.

To begin with, this type of organ donation is often based on a response to patients advertising their need for an organ donor publicly via billboards, television, or the Internet. Although not illegal, some contend that this approach undermines the laws that organs cannot be bought or sold. People who can afford to advertise for an organ, critics point out, have an unfair advantage over poorer people who cannot. For example, the monthly subscription fee for a patient to be listed on one Web site for matching patients with people willing to be living donors is approximately $300.

Critics opposed to advertising for living donors also point out that advertising bypasses the fair waiting system set up by UNOS and can lead to organs being "wasted." In one case, a Texas man dying from a liver disease advertised for and found a living donor. However, he died within a year of receiving the transplant anyway. Although volunteer living donors that participate in efforts such as MatchingDonors.com do not receive payment for their organs, they are reimbursed for expenses, such as travel, housing, and meals. Some fear that such an approach to obtaining organs will ultimately subvert the entire process, leading to illegal payments for organs because people with enough money can often find their way around such prohibitions.

Yet another argument against advertising for living donors is that people who can present the most compelling stories are also the ones likely to get a living donor organ through such programs. Placing an advertisement with a picture of a young, pretty, curly-haired little girl with an emotional plea from her parents is far more likely to elicit a response than an ad featuring a former alcoholic or even ads featuring older people in general. Some argue that, when solicitation is allowed, the entire process gets skewed in favor of those who are able to make the most noise and the best pleas. This ability, however, does not necessarily mean that they are most deserving of a transplant, which is primarily a subjective value judgment at best. Also, they argue, Internet programs for soliciting organs do not do a good job of screening donors either in terms of donors' competency or in terms of informed consent.

Allowing living donors to "select" which strangers they want to give their organs to also opens up questions about some donors possibly choosing recipients on the basis of race, religion, or ethnicity. Opponents point out that allowing donors to choose strangers is ultimately unfair because it would be nearly impossible to factor out such discriminatory aspects. For example, although the case involved a cadaveric donor, a family in Florida tried to stipulate that the donor's organs could not go to blacks because the donor had been a racist his whole life and would not have wanted a black person to receive any of his organs.

Those in favor of programs such as Internet sites that allow patients to advertise for living donors argue that, in a free society, it is an individual's right to choose whom they want to give an organ to, just like they can vote for whomever they like and give to the charities of their choice. Proponents also point out that they believe that directed donations to strangers leads to the availability of organs that might otherwise not have been donated. Not only does this scenario not harm anyone, they argue, but it actually decreases the need for organ donors because these recipients are removed from the donor organ waiting list.

Another argument in favor of the practice is that the UNOS system for procuring cadaveric donors also is unfair in that organs can be stipulated to be donated locally within the donor's specific region. Proponents of allowing directed living donations contend that people who are wealthy and knowledgeable about the UNOS system gain an unfair advantage because they can get on several regional lists. Furthermore, some argue that the UNOS system is for cadaveric, or dead, donors, whereas advertising can take place only for living donors. Thus, the likelihood of undermining the UNOS system is minimal. Finally, proponents ask those who oppose advertising for donors this question: is it more ethical to let people die while waiting for an organ?

Few believe that the solicitation of organs over the Internet and other venues will ever stop or that living donations will be halted because of risks to the donor. For example, many think that partial lung and pancreas transplants may increase significantly as surgical techniques for these procedures improve. Many observers also contend that some type of nationwide system should be set up similar to the UNOS system to help regulate and control the allocation of organs by living donors to strangers. In addition, there is a growing effort to establish a strong follow-up data-gathering system to determine just what long-term effects living donation has on the donors over the years. In fact, the National Institutes of Health has begun a seven-year research study focusing on living donors at nine transplant centers throughout the United States.

To many, leaving decisions about living donations up to the transplant centers is problematic because organ transplantation is big business, which lends itself to abuse. Ultimately, as living donor transplants increase, both transplant centers and government will likely work together to ensure that a proper registry is established for living donors and that uniform standards are set in the United States. Efforts are also underway to ensure that living donors are protected by advocates who have no monetary or other interest in the process. For example, a group of nurses and others have already established the Living Organ Donor Advocate Program (LODAP), which provides nurse advocates for living donors. LODAP is also proposing that the federal government pass legislation that would establish both a federally funded National Donor Advocate Agency and a National Registry for Living Organ Donors.

CHAPTER 9

Stem Cell Transplantation and Research: A Question of Life?

In his 1932 classic novel *A Brave New World*, Aldous Huxley described a future in which "hatcheries" produced human beings created in test tubes. Less than fifty years later, Huxley's vision materialized with the late 1970s development of in vitro fertilization to help infertile couples become pregnant. This reproductive assistive technology combines a man's sperm and a woman's egg in a laboratory and then transfers the resulting embryo into the woman's uterus or womb, where it can develop naturally. To help ensure success, several embryos may be placed in the woman's uterus at one time. Often referred to as "test tube babies," more than a quarter of a million children have been born using this technique.

Although some controversy has surrounded in vitro fertilization, the public has largely accepted it as a viable alternative to natural pregnancy. At one time, the public gave little thought to in vitro fertilization and did not realize that clinics routinely create many eggs or embryos so that more will be available in case the woman fails to become pregnant with the first implant. As a result of this practice, the number of embryos stored in liquid nitrogen in clinics throughout the United States alone is estimated at 400,000 (Weiss, 2003, p. A10).

These stored embryos may have remained for the most part forgotten if not for a growing research effort involving embryonic stem cells—immature, uniform cells that can differentiate or evolve into any kind of cell and tissue. Research that began in the 1990s has led to what may be one of the most monumental advances in medical science since the development of antibiotics: the transplantation of microscopic cells to treat a wide variety of diseases and other medical problems. It has also engendered a heated debate involving science, religion, politics, and an estimated two billion people around the world with medical problems ranging from Parkinson's and Alzheimer's disease to diabetes, heart disease, and cancer (see the Chapter 4 section on stem cells). Overall, it is estimated that 100 to 200 million people may suffer from chronic degenerative and acute diseases that stem cell transplantation may one day be able to treat.

Although research with fully mature stem cells found in adults has shown some promise, many scientists believe that the greatest potential involves transplanting embryonic stem cells into specific parts of the body, where they can grow and develop into functioning cells and tissue to treat a variety of diseases and medical problems. Although the research is still in its relative infancy, some medical scientists see a bright future for embryonic stem cell transplantation. One of the primary resources for gathering embryonic stem cells is the storage vaults of in vitro fertilization clinics. Other sources include aborted fetuses. Efforts are also underway to clone human embryos as sources of stem cells for research, and scientists at the Jones Institute in Virginia have mixed sperm and eggs for the sole purpose of creating embryos to provide stem cells for scientific study.

Embryonic stem cell transplantation has sparked one of the biggest debates in modern medical research. The controversy revolves around the fact that taking stem cells from embryos results in their destruction. As a result, using these cells for research leads to questions of when life begins and whether the "death" of an embryo is morally justified or essentially the murder of a potential human being.

THE PRESIDENT TAKES A STAND

The political and governmental stance on research involving the use of either fetal tissue or human embryos began in the early 1980s with a ban on federal funding for research involving either fetal tissue or embryos. Nearly twenty years later, advancing research into stem cells raised the stakes as scientists produced new evidence that embryonic stem cells could one day be used to treat millions of people in the United States and billions around the world.

On August 9, 2001, President George W. Bush addressed the nation concerning embryonic stem cell research. In a televised speech, the president referred to the Jones Institute's use of in vitro fertilization techniques to create "experimental" embryos, noting, "In recent weeks, we learned that scientists have created human embryos in test tubes solely to experiment on them. This is deeply troubling, and a warning sign that should prompt all of us to think through these issues very carefully" (Bush, 2001). He went on to state that under his presidency, the federal government's policy for funding embryonic stem cell research would be limited to the approximately seventy stem cell lines (a reservoir of cells derived from a single embryo) in existence that had already been created from the embryos destroyed by clinics. Bush further proposed support for more aggressive funding into research with animal and adult stem cells, such as stem cells gathered from umbilical cords, bone marrow, and fat. The president noted, "This allows us to explore the promise and potential of stem cell research without crossing a fundamental moral line, by providing taxpayer funding that would sanction or encourage further destruction of human embryos that have at least the potential for life" (Bush, 2001).

On the surface, Bush's stance seemed to be a politically safe position that would allow continued research and avoid the growing ethical dilemma involving embryonic stem cell research. In reality, the president's address brought the issue under even more political and public scrutiny. U.S. researchers could still use private funding for research, but the scientific community noted that government support was the only way to get enough funds to comprehensively conduct such research and put it on a fast pace to save lives and improve quality of life. Furthermore, it became increasingly clear that the available stem cell lines, which were thought to have the ability to regenerate themselves indefinitely, were actually degrading, so that by 2006 it was estimated that possibly only about ten, if any, of these lines were still suitable for research.

The debate over embryonic stem cell research is not limited to the United States. Although some governments, such as Great Britain and Australia, support research in this area, others, such as Italy, Germany, Austria, Portugal, Spain, and Ireland, have established laws opposing such efforts and banning government funding for them. In 2006, a meeting of the European Union failed to establish an agreed-upon set of principles guiding embryonic stem cell research for its member nations.

EMBRYONIC STEM CELLS AND THE "SANCTITY OF LIFE"

The controversy surrounding embryonic stem cell research and transplantation is closely tied with the ethical conflict over abortion and is similarly highly charged. On one side are direly ill patients, their families, many scientists, and those in the general public who agree with them that it is unfair to deny living human beings a chance for a longer and better life because of the destruction of a microscopic cluster of cells. At best, they contend, these cells are like skin and other human tissue, which in and of themselves do not constitute a human life.

On the other side are those who argue that these embryonic cells have the potential to become a human life and, as a result, deserve the same respect as a child or an adult. Sacrificing one life to save another, they believe, is morally wrong and reprehensible. The most zealous opponents have compared embryonic stem cell research to Nazi experiments with humans during World War II, which resulted in such atrocities as making lamp shades out of human skin.

At the root of the issue, however, is the question "When does life begin?" Unfortunately, as the abortion debate has shown, reaching a consensus about when human "life" begins may never be resolved. Those who oppose using embryonic stem cells believe that life begins at conception. For opponents, or "pro-lifers," it doesn't matter whether the embryo was conceived naturally or in a petri dish in a lab. As for all of the stored embryos, opponents of stem cell research believe that these embryos could, at some point, be implanted into a woman's uterus and grow into a human being. Furthermore, many of those who are religious argue that these embryos, in a sense, have already received a soul, further bolstering in their eyes the argument that destroying theses embryos constitutes murder.

Proponents of embryonic stem cell research believe that there is an approach that may sidestep the "potential human being" argument against embryonic stem cell research. Altered nuclear transfer, or ANT, is a process that involves creating genetically-altered embryos that are not suitable for implantation into a uterus, and then extracting stem cells from these unusable embryos. Given that these cells cannot become a viable embryo that could produce life, proponents claim that they should not be considered "potential" human lives.

Those who favor embryonic stem cell research and transplantation are similar in their beliefs to those on the "pro-choice" side of the abortion debate. They consider these masses of cells not to constitute a person until much later in their maturation and growth, either during the later fetal stages of pregnancy or perhaps at birth when the fetus is separated from his or her mother.

Although no consensus has been reached about when personhood begins, in its most basic state, human life can be defined as any living entity that contains human DNA. As a result, spermatozoa, a woman's ovum, an egg at the moment of fertilization, and an embryo consisting of differentiated cells can all be considered forms of human life. Even a pre-embryo, according to the view of some, has the "potentiality" to become a person.

Life and Personhood: Some Scientific Perspectives

The debate over when human life, or personhood, begins dates back thousands of years, and there are many viewpoints concerning this issue associated with religions and cultures. The following are some science-based perspectives on when human "life" may begin.

Metabolic view: No single moment marks the beginning of human life. Because both sperm and egg cells can individually be considered units of life, the beginning of new life cannot be designated as either the union of two gametes (a mature sexual reproductive cell that has one set of unpaired chromosomes) or any other developmental point. Also encompassed within a "metabolic" viewpoint of life is the idea that marking points such as the fourteen-day division between a zygote and an embryo are artificial constructions used by biologists and doctors for categorization purposes.

Genetic view: Fertilization marks the beginning of human life because it is when genetic material combines to make a unique individual.

Embryological view: Human life originates at gastrulation, that is, when the process of forming a gastrula begins. Gastrula is the double-walled stage of the embryo that involves the beginning of cell movements by which a developing embryo forms distinct layers that later grow into different organs.

Neurological view: Human life begins at the time a fetus has a recognizable EEG (electroencephalogram) pattern, which occurs at approximately twenty-four to twenty-seven weeks after conception of the fetus. This is the point at which brain activity can be described as characteristically human.

A "pre-embryo" can be defined as a ball of about 150 cells that develop from a fertilized egg but have not yet attached to the uterus lining to form a full embryo. In the pre-embryonic state, these cells have yet to differentiate and have no brain, central nervous system, or internal organs. Embryonic stem cells are taken from the pre-embryonic ball of cells. Some argue, however, that "pre-embryonic" is an "artificial" term created as part of a rationale for permitting human embryo research.

Those in favor of embryonic research, however, note that potential for life is not life. They argue that people are not worried about the loss of human DNA when men ejaculate and thousands of spermatozoa enter the woman's body but are eventually rejected in the form of an unfertilized egg. Birth control, they point out, is also stopping the "potential" for life by preventing pregnancy. For example, the use of intra-uterine devices (IUDs) is

---

Embryo Adoption

In 1997 the Snowflakes Embryo Adoption Program was established in collaboration with the Nightlight Christian Adoptions. According to the program, "snowflakes" was chosen as part of the name to reflect the unique and fragile state of human embryos. Although there is some question as to why people would consider embryo adoption, which must be approved by the original "parents," supporters point out that it is less expensive than other similar approaches such as egg donation, and it enables the couple to experience pregnancy and ensure good prenatal care. The federal government under George W. Bush has for the first time made federal funding available for Snowflakes and other embryo adoption programs and for raising public awareness about this option. There are risks to the embryo during the adoption process. Only about half the embryos donated survive the thawing process. Of those that do survive, a little more than one-third result in a child. Although no concrete statistics exist on exactly how many embryo adoptions have occurred throughout the United States, a 2003 survey by the American Society for Reproductive Medicine found that about 2 percent of the possibly 400,000 frozen embryos in existence have been given to other families.

---

believed to result in millions of deaths of fertilized embryos each year in North America, much more than those killed by surgical abortions. Yet, they argue, few pro-life efforts have focused on stopping the use of IUDs.

Though religious organizations such as the Catholic Church do oppose birth control, the vast majority of the general public and many religions do not oppose most birth control methods that prevent initial pregnancy. Nevertheless, some argue that the embryo, or pre-embryo, should be respected. Even thought it is not assigned the status of a human person, they contend that it is a step closer to personhood than the cells in an ovum or spermatozoa and, thus, has greater potential to become a human being.

Another argument cited by those in favor of embryonic stem cell research is that many of the embryos already stored at in vitro fertilization clinics will eventually be destroyed and that not using them for research is a waste. Opponents contend that these embryos should be viewed as "frozen orphanages," where embryos can be stored for eventual adoption by people who want to have children. Such "adoptions," they say, would save "lives." They point out that using these stored embryos could be more satisfying for some than adopting already-born children because the mother and father would go through the entire pregnancy process, establishing an even stronger bond with the child.

WHO'S ON WHOSE SIDE?

Although the debate over stem cell research in many ways is similar to the abortion debate, not all "pro-lifers" are against embryonic stem cell research. Many, in fact, have sided with the scientific community and favor continuing research and government funding for it. For example, staunch conservative politicians such as Republican senators Orrin Hatch and Bill Frist, a former transplant surgeon, have come out in favor of the research, siding with science and high-profile people who suffer from diseases that may be treated one day with the approach, such as Parkinson's disease patient and actor Michael J. Fox. In January 2004, fifty-eight U.S. senators, including fourteen Republicans, wrote a letter to Bush in favor of using spare frozen embryos for stem cell research.

The issue was also part of the 2004 U.S. presidential election, with Bush's opponent Senator John Kerry in favor of the research and Bush opposed to it. The distinction between conservatives and liberals and pro-lifers and those who are pro-choice in the abortion debate was further clouded concerning embryonic stem cell research when people like Nancy Reagan, wife of former conservative President Ronald Reagan, came out in favor of the research. Many have touted stem cells as a potential treatment for Alzeheimer's disease, which afflicted the late president.

Several polls have indicated that the majority of the U.S. population supports embryonic stem cell research, including many staunchly conservative Republican voters. For example, a 2001 poll conducted by TNS Intersearch for ABC News, found that Americans supported stem cell research and federal funding for it by approximately a two-to-one margin, including Catholics (Langer, 2001). Another poll by Caravan OCR International for the Coalition for the Advancement of Medical Research, found that 70 percent of the people polled favored the research. Interestingly, even fundamentalist Christians supported the research by a 2.5-to-1 margin, and 56 percent of people who identified themselves as pro-lifers favored efforts in this area (Coalition for the Advancement of Medical Research, 2001).

Finally, although women's rights activists have generally not been on the pro-life side of the abortion debate, some have come out against the idea of using embryonic stem cells for research. Along with other opponents, they fear that women's essential rights may be abused by the creation of "egg farms" for research. They note that the need for human

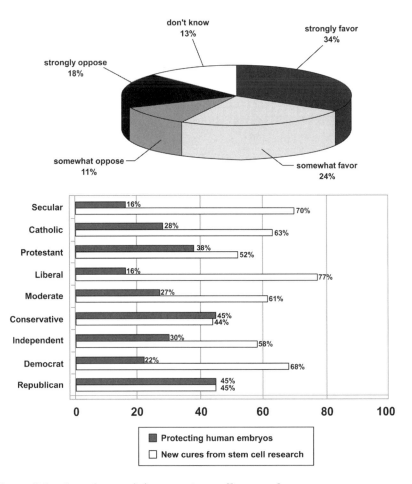

Figure 9.1   American opinions on stem cell research
Almost every poll focusing on a broad cross section of the American public has
found that people in general favor embryonic stem cell research. The pie chart
shows the results of The Parade/Research! America Health Poll, Charlton
Research Company, conducted in 2005. Overall, 58% of Americans either
"strongly" or "somewhat" favor embryonic stem cell research whereas only 29%
"somewhat" or "strongly" oppose (Research America, 2005).

The bar graph reveals how opinions about stem cell research vary along religious and political lines. The graph comes from data gathered from a 2004 poll of
2,000 adults conducted by the Pew Research Center for the People and the Press,
which was published in a press release in 2005. It illustrates answers, by group-
ings, to the question "Which are more important?" with the answer choices being
"New cures from stem cell research" (represented by the white bar) and "Protect-
ing human embryos" (represented by the shaded bar) (Pew Research Center for
the People and the Press, 2005).

> **California Skirts Opposition and Hands Out Stem Cell Grants**
>
> Although California passed legislation in 2004 to fund stem cell research, the program remained in limbo because of numerous lawsuits by groups opposing such research. These suits have prevented the state from distributing any of the $3 billion in tax dollars appropriated for the research funding. In April 2006, the state temporarily sidestepped the issue and handed out its first round of grants using money supplied by state business leaders who bought "bond anticipation notes," a type of loan, to support the funding. Many were pleased with the state's efforts to start funding embryonic stem cell research, but some in favor of such research were concerned that the private investors could unduly influence the research activities.

embryos could lead to a potentially lucrative market in human eggs that could put women at risk of exploitation.

As for the federal ban on embryonic stem cell research using new cell lines, some states have voiced their different views by passing laws allowing such research and the use of state tax monies to support the efforts. In January 2003, California Bill SB 253 took effect authorizing such research and devoting $3 billion in state tax dollars in the form of bonds approved by voters to fund it. New Jersey became the second state to permit publicly funded research with embryonic stem cells in January of the following year.

ADULT STEM CELLS: A VIABLE ALTERNATIVE?

An article in a January 2002 issue of the *New Scientist* reported that a University of Minnesota team had discovered stem cells (called multipotent adult progenitor cells, or MAPCs) in the bone marrow of adults that showed potential for developing into almost any of the 220 tissue types found in the human body. However, this research is at the early stages, and questions remain about whether MAPCs can form functioning human cells. Furthermore, studies on the use of adult stem cells and their ability to transform themselves into such things as heart muscle have not been replicated. Nevertheless, another approach being developed at the University of Pittsburgh involves the discovery and use of cells in human placentas that are similar to embryonic stem cells.

Those in favor of using embryonic stem cells for research and transplantation point out that trying to use adult stem cells has many limitations not associated with embryonic stem cells and, as a result, may have limited potential for therapeutic use. They note that researchers have not yet found stem cells in adults that could become all cell and tissue types found in the human body, such as pancreatic islet cells, which have yet to be identified in adult humans. Furthermore, adult stem cells are usually present in very small numbers and are difficult to isolate and purify. It is also believed that the number of these cells may decrease with age. Some also argue that the jury remains out on the promise of these cells whereas embryonic stem cells are generally believed to have a much greater potential for being developed into viable therapies.

Some scientists who favor embryonic stem cell research fear that advances with adult stem cells may hinder embryonic stem cell research because it can be used as an argument against these efforts. They point out that there are still important biological differences between adult and embryonic stem cells. Despite the enthusiasm generated by some research results, the potential for adult stem cells to actually differentiate into other cell types is uncertain. On the other hand, human embryonic stem cells, they say, have clearly shown their ability to develop into multiple tissue types. Furthermore, they exhibit long-term self-renewal in cultures, something scientists are having a difficult time achieving with adult cells.

NOT A SURE THING

Although many scientists believe embryonic stem cell research holds much promise, there are also those within the scientific community who are skeptical. No foolproof, successful therapy has yet been developed, and many question whether immune system barriers can be overcome to ensure that the cells won't be rejected. Furthermore, there is no guarantee that these cells will ever integrate with their new host and form functioning tissue. Some are also concerned about these transplanted cells' potential to "overgrow," a process associated with certain types of cancers.

There is little doubt that emotions run high in the arguments for and against embryonic stem cell research. The conflicting ethical perspectives that surround the use of these cells in humans go to the core of opposing beliefs. In the end, opinions about whether research should go forward using embryonic stem cells remains tied to an individual's belief about the status of human embryos. For those against embryonic stem cell research, the moral price is a far too high price to pay for any potential benefits. For scientists and many families of people with chronic and degenerative diseases that may one day be cured, or at the very least alleviated, by stem cell transplants, to stop research would be ignoring a medical boon for humankind.

Although conflicting ethical perspectives have resulted in a heated debate over embryonic stem cell research, scientists point out that this is not the first debate of its kind related to biomedical research. In the past, as in the case of recombinant DNA research, the government has stepped in and set high scientific and ethical standards for conducting such research. If embryonic stem cell research is to continue and garner federal funding, government organizations such as the National Institutes of Health likely will establish similar standards for embryonic stem cell research while ensuring that any proposal of research in this area is scientifically justified.

CHAPTER 10

Face Transplants: Some Ethical Considerations

Despite the teaching that "it is what's inside that counts," few would dispute that our appearance plays a crucial role in our sense of self and in how others perceive us. How important is our appearance? One indicator of society's emphasis on "looks" is that plastic surgery has become the fastest-growing surgical field today as people have their chins, noses, eyes, and cheekbones reshaped to fit to some perceived notion of the ideal. It is little wonder then that people who suffer from facial disfigurements can experience extreme emotional and psychological difficulties.

The promise of face transplants became a reality by the end of the 1990s when scientists, through the use of immunosuppressive drugs, began to overcome the strong immune system barrier that has largely prevented successful skin grafts between two individuals who are not identical twins. Unlike cosmetic surgery, skin grafts and face transplantations are being researched to help people with severe facial disfigurements. Potential candidates for face transplants include burn and trauma victims and people suffering from disfiguring head and neck cancers. (Because face transplants do not include restructuring bone and cartilage, the procedure may not apply to such problems as disfiguring congenital defects.) Although the technology and procedures to perform a face transplant are several years old, surgeons and medical centers have been reluctant to attempt the procedure because of a complex set of medical and ethical questions.

For the most part, the ethical concerns over face transplants remained largely within the medical and ethical communities. Recent developments, however, have propelled face transplantation into the headlines along with several debates concerning the procedure. Surgeons in France completed the first partial face transplant in 2005 on a woman who had been disfigured by a dog attack (see sidebar). Then, in March of 2006, plastic surgeons at the Cleveland Clinic announced that their research with cadavers had produced a promising approach for a complete face transplant.

Much of the medical community and many others perceive face transplants as offering new hope for thousands of people suffering from facial disfigurement. The procedure has the potential to transform these patients' lives, allowing many people who have literally shut themselves off from the world to once again venture forth and interact with others without the social stigma of a disfigured appearance. Critics, however, have expressed several concerns about performing face transplants. Are the benefits worth the long-term medical risks? Considering the experimental nature of the procedure, can a prospective patient truly make a decision based on informed consent? What are the potential psychological ramifications?

First Partial Face Transplant and Ethical Questions

The first partial face transplant occurred in France in 2005 and raised the eyebrows of both medical professionals and ethicists. For example, the surgeons also used another experimental technique of including a bone marrow transplant to help prevent rejection. Adding a second experimental procedure to the first is not considered good practice in experimental procedures performed on humans and may make it difficult to determine down the road why the experiment succeeded or failed. Furthermore, some questioned the recipient's psychological competence to undergo such a procedure given that she had reportedly tried to commit suicide even before the disfiguring accident. Some were concerned that the medical team did not seem interested in trying more standard approaches to repair the women's face but instead rushed into the face transplant procedure, raising questions about the physicians' motives. Were they operating in the best interest of the patient, or were they out to gain recognition as "the first" to perform such a transplant? Many were also troubled by the fact that the recipient had made a financial deal with British moviemakers for the rights to her story. Another concern was the leaking of the donor's and the transplant recipient's identities, especially in light of the intense media attention garnered and the potential psychological repercussions of such attention on the recipient and the donor family.

Some have referred to face transplantation as "a grand human experiment." However, the procedure is surgically, immunologically, and psychologically complicated with uncertain outcomes and impacts on the transplant recipient. Although few would deny the potential benefits of face transplantation, careful examination of the issue reveals that there is more to the procedure than meets the eye.

LONG-TERM RISKS AND INFORMED CONSENT

Like almost all types of transplants, face transplantation will require that patients undergo an intensive regimen of immunosuppressive therapy for the remainder of their lives. Immunosuppression in transplantation comes with many long-term risks, including the potential to develop cancer, kidney failure, infections, diabetes, and high blood pressure, all of which can be life-threatening. Many critics of face transplants argue that these risks are far too great for a procedure that, unlike organ transplantation, is not necessary to save the patient's life. In the mind of some, the negative impact that these complications could have on patients potentially outweighs the promised, but as yet unproven, benefits of a procedure that may never provide a functioning or partially functioning face.

Another concern is that the procedure is so new and experimental that potential patients may not be able to make a reasonable judgment based on informed consent about whether to undergo the procedure. In fact, until more research is performed, especially in animals, many critics believe that informed consent is virtually impossible. For example, no one can predict or provide statistical analysis relating to potential complications, including infections that could turn the recipient's new face black and require a second transplant or skin graft reconstruction. Some argue that those who might opt for such a highly experimental and high-risk procedure are already emotionally fragile because of their disfigurement. Skeptics believe that these are the people who are least likely to cope effectively with bad results that may leave them worse off than before.

Despite these problems, proponents of face transplants point out that potential recipients have the right to make these decisions based on the information available. This information is primarily a "best guess" scenario based on results from other types of transplants, including a limited number of hand transplants performed around the world. According to a 2004 report by England's Royal College of Surgeons, the rate of acute rejection of a face transplant within one year may be approximately 10 percent, and chronic rejection over a longer period could be as high as 30 to 50 percent.

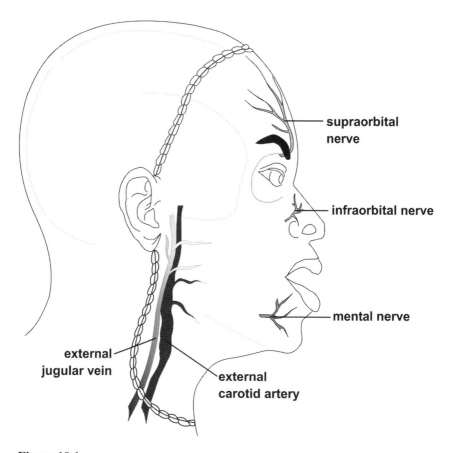

Figure 10.1
The above illustration shows how a total facial transplant might be sutured into place,
where the corresponding vessels of the graft and the supraorbital, infraorbital, and
mental nerves on each side might be connected to provide sensation and functioning.

Scientists currently researching or preparing to perform such transplants note that informed consent forms indicate that the potential for these
risks is unknown and potentially very high. Nevertheless, researchers
report that they have had many people with disfigurements contact them,
indicating that they are more than willing to take such risks and be "pioneers" for a chance to once again lead a full and active life. For example,
researchers at the University of Louisville seeking to perform a full face
transplant have conducted research with questionnaires that included que-
ries about how many years of life expectancy they would be willing to give
up for a transplanted organ. Preliminary results have varied depending on

the organ or body part. For example, more people were willing to give up more years of life for a larynx than for a hand. Perhaps not surprising is the fact that "the body part for which people are willing to trade most years of life is by some margin a transplanted face" (Concar, 2004, p. 32).

Although face transplants may not be a literal life-or-death situation, proponents of face transplantation contend that people with severe facial disfigurements face a risk of committing suicide that is around four times higher than the general population. In a sense, some are "metaphorically" dead in terms of encountering severe depression and having an extremely poor quality of life that often includes a lack of companionship, meaningful employment, and other aspects that lead to social well-being. Some stress that the situation is similar to many other procedures once considered experimental. They point to the early days of organ transplantation as an example of the value of gaining comprehensive data through experience.

Although all surgeries contain inherent risks, such as the chance of infection, some believe that face transplantation may have less chance of complications than current skin-grafting methods used to repair faces. Sometimes, skin-graft patients may undergo as many as forty or fifty operations with mixed results and often only limited function, making skin grafts an unsatisfactory alternative to face transplants. In the case of face transplants, they contend that the texture and pliability of facial skin can be matched to a much higher degree than skin grafts.

A CASE OF IDENTITY

Another issue surrounding face transplants is the recipients' sense of identity. Our face is undoubtedly our most identifying feature and is also how we often express ourselves without the use of words. A smile, a frown, or a raised eyebrow can reveal in a flash what we are thinking and bestow upon others our sense of approval and love or consternation and condemnation. Although face transplantation may offer the best hope for repairing such functioning to the face, no one can predict how people will respond to what ultimately appears to be a new identity.

If full functioning—that is, the ability to express emotions through manipulation of facial features—does not return to the face, skeptics argue that the recipient may end up with little more than a "mask." Research has also shown that even donor organ recipients have reported ambivalent or negative feelings about having another person's organ keep them alive. Having a new face would only intensify such feelings, many contend. Those who urge caution with this procedure point to the case of a man who received a hand transplant but could not fully identify with the hand as being part of his body and ultimately quit taking his immunosuppressive medications, resulting in the hand's removal. Furthermore, not only will recipients have to face a new physical identity when they look in the mirror, but they also will have to deal with the reaction of their family and friends, who may react to them quite differently.

Despite these considerations, some observers point out that people with severe facial disfigurements already have been dealing with a loss of identity and often face extremely negative reactions from others because of their disfigurement. Furthermore, identity, they contend, is more strongly associated with personality than with facial appearances, especially in terms of friends, family, and others who know someone. They stress that having a more normal appearance, even if it isn't fully functional, can only be an improvement for extremely disfigured patients. Of course, each individual will react somewhat differently, and some will be able to handle the stresses and psychological impact better than others.

Many of the identity difficulties, proponents of moving forward with face transplants contend, can be mitigated by ongoing psychological counseling. They also point out that face-transplant recipients will still have their own eyes, which, as the saying goes, are the "window to the soul." Supporters argue that although the concept of identity is linked to a person's facial appearance, surgeons in fact are not transplanting identity but merely facial tissue, which the recipient and those around them can probably adjust to much more easily than they can to disfigurement.

WHO WILL GET A FACE?

Although face transplantation is still in the early experimental stages and far from becoming a routine procedure, ethicists are already pondering the impact of the procedure if it becomes a success and is performed on a widespread basis. As success in organ transplantation has shown, getting enough donor organs to fill the need has been one of the field's most controversial and problematic aspects. If individuals and their families are reluctant to donate organs, how much more reluctant will they be to donate a part of a person so identifiable as a face? Although the person who receives the transplanted face will not look like the deceased because of underlying bone structure and muscles unique to each individual, donating a face is likely to involve even more of a psychological barrier than donating organs because the face is the most "symbolic" representation of a person. Furthermore, part of the grieving process traditionally involves open caskets for viewing by friends and relatives. Because the face would have to be removed at the time of death, family and friends may not be able to partake in this ritual. (In the case of the donor for the partial face transplant in France, a "mask" of the donor's face was constructed for funeral purposes.)

Also limiting the availability of donor faces is the fact that most people do not die under conditions that would enable their face, or other organs for that matter, to be harvested. In addition, unlike donor organs, donor faces would likely have to be matched both in color and in gender.

Because of the likelihood that not enough donor faces will be available to fulfill need, the question of allocation once again comes to the forefront of transplantation. How will it be determined who can receive the limited number of faces available for transplant? Will it depend on how well a person is able to cope with their current deformity? What role will economic factors play, such as the ability of the person to pay for the long-term use of expensive immunosuppressive medications that can cost $10,000 to $12,000 a year?

Both the proponents and opponents to quickly advancing face-transplant experiments on humans recognize the ethical dilemmas surrounding the procedure. They also agree that some arguments against it, such as the likelihood of it becoming a cosmetic procedure, are highly unlikely considering the risks involved.

Although ethical concerns exist, face transplantation is likely to advance for the simple reason that it offers the potential for a vast improvement in the quality of life for extremely disfigured people. Throughout the field's history, transplant professionals have pushed the envelope. In balancing the risk and the benefits of face transplants, researchers, patients, and the general public will have to further examine the consequences of this breakthrough that involves a part of the human body inextricably linked with a person's identity. Both sides also caution that patients will have to have realistic expectations about the outcome and the cosmetic improvements, which are unlikely to match the ideal.

References and Resources

APPENDIX A

Annotated Primary Source Documents

APPENDIX ITEM I: PRESIDENT GEORGE W. BUSH'S SPEECH ON STEM CELL RESEARCH

Chapter 9 in *Organ Transplantation* discusses the issues surrounding stem cell research, including the official stance of the U.S. Government on stem cell research involving the use of embryonic stem cells. The following is a speech given by President George W. Bush concerning his beliefs about the appropriateness of stem cell research. In May 2001, prior to giving this speech the following August, President Bush banned the use of federal funds for stem cell research using embryonic stem cell lines that were not already in existence. This "official" stance has led to a groundswell of controversy, including many Republican officials within the president's own party disagreeing with the President's decision in this matter. For example, then majority leader and ultra-conservative Senator Bill Frist broke from the White House in this matter to come out in support of a bill to provide funding for embryonic stem cell research, which many in the medical community believe holds vast promise for treating numerous diseases that have proved resistant to other medical approaches and treatments. This speech can also be accessed at the White House Web site at http://www.whitehouse.gov/news/releases/2001/08/20010809-2.html.

For Immediate Release
Office of the Press Secretary
August 9, 2001
President Discusses Stem Cell Research
The Bush Ranch, Crawford, Texas
8:01 P.M. CDT

THE PRESIDENT: Good evening. I appreciate you giving me a few minutes of your time tonight so I can discuss with you a complex and difficult issue, an issue that is one of the most profound of our time.

The issue of research involving stem cells derived from human embryos is increasingly the subject of a national debate and dinner table discussions. The issue is confronted every day in laboratories as scientists ponder the ethical ramifications of their work. It is agonized over by parents and many couples as they try to have children, or to save children already born.

The issue is debated within the church, with people of different faiths, even many of the same faith coming to different conclusions. Many people are finding that the more they know about stem cell research, the less certain they are about the right ethical and moral conclusions.

My administration must decide whether to allow federal funds, your tax dollars, to be used for scientific research on stem cells derived from human embryos. A large number of these embryos already exist. They are the product of a process called in vitro fertilization, which helps so many couples conceive children. When doctors match sperm and egg to create life outside the womb, they usually produce more embryos than are planted in the mother. Once a couple successfully has children, or if they are unsuccessful, the additional embryos remain frozen in laboratories.

Some will not survive during long storage; others are destroyed. A number have been donated to science and used to create privately funded stem cell lines. And a few have been implanted in an adoptive mother and born, and are today healthy children.

Based on preliminary work that has been privately funded, scientists believe further research using stem cells offers great promise that could help improve the lives of those who suffer from many terrible diseases—from juvenile diabetes to Alzheimer's, from Parkinson's to spinal cord injuries. And while scientists admit they are not yet certain, they believe stem cells derived from embryos have unique potential.

You should also know that stem cells can be derived from sources other than embryos—from adult cells, from umbilical cords that are discarded after babies are born, from human placenta. And many scientists feel research on these types of stem cells is also promising. Many patients suffering from a range of diseases are already being helped with treatments developed from adult stem cells.

However, most scientists, at least today, believe that research on embryonic stem cells offers the most promise because these cells have the potential to develop in all of the tissues in the body.

Scientists further believe that rapid progress in this research will come only with federal funds. Federal dollars help attract the best and brightest scientists. They ensure new discoveries are widely shared at the largest number of research facilities and that the research is directed toward the greatest public good.

The United States has a long and proud record of leading the world toward advances in science and medicine that improve human life. And the United States has a long and proud record of upholding the highest standards of ethics as we expand the limits of science and knowledge. Research on embryonic stem cells raises profound ethical questions, because extracting the stem cell destroys the embryo, and thus destroys its potential for life. Like a snowflake, each of these embryos is unique, with the unique genetic potential of an individual human being.

As I thought through this issue, I kept returning to two fundamental questions: First, are these frozen embryos human life, and therefore, something precious to be protected? And second, if they're going to be destroyed anyway, shouldn't they be used for a greater good, for research that has the potential to save and improve other lives?

I've asked those questions and others of scientists, scholars, bioethicists, religious leaders, doctors, researchers, members of Congress, my Cabinet, and my friends. I have read heartfelt letters from many Americans. I have given this issue a great deal of thought, prayer and considerable reflection. And I have found widespread disagreement.

On the first issue, are these embryos human life—well, one researcher told me he believes this five-day-old cluster of cells is not an embryo, not yet an individual, but a pre-embryo. He argued that it has the potential for life, but it is not a life because it cannot develop on its own.

An ethicist dismissed that as a callous attempt at rationalization. Make no mistake, he told me, that cluster of cells is the same way you and I, and all the rest of us, started our lives. One goes with a heavy heart if we use these, he said, because we are dealing with the seeds of the next generation.

And to the other crucial question, if these are going to be destroyed any-way, why not use them for good purpose—I also found different answers. Many argue these embryos are byproducts of a process that helps create life, and we should allow couples to donate them to science so they can be used for good purpose instead of wasting their potential. Others will argue there's no such thing as excess life, and the fact that a living being is going to die does not justify experimenting on it or exploiting it as a natural resource.

At its core, this issue forces us to confront fundamental questions about the beginnings of life and the ends of science. It lies at a difficult moral intersection, juxtaposing the need to protect life in all its phases with the prospect of saving and improving life in all its stages.

As the discoveries of modern science create tremendous hope, they also lay vast ethical mine fields. As the genius of science extends the horizons of what we can do, we increasingly confront complex questions about what we should do. We have arrived at that brave new world that seemed so distant in 1932, when Aldous Huxley wrote about human beings created in test tubes in what he called a "hatchery."

In recent weeks, we learned that scientists have created human embryos in test tubes solely to experiment on them. This is deeply trou-bling, and a warning sign that should prompt all of us to think through these issues very carefully.

Embryonic stem cell research is at the leading edge of a series of moral hazards. The initial stem cell researcher was at first reluctant to begin his research, fearing it might be used for human cloning. Scien-tists have already cloned a sheep. Researchers are telling us the next step could be to clone human beings to create individual designer stem cells, essentially to grow another you, to be available in case you need another heart or lung or liver.

I strongly oppose human cloning, as do most Americans. We recoil at the idea of growing human beings for spare body parts, or creating life for our convenience. And while we must devote enormous energy to conquering disease, it is equally important that we pay attention to the moral concerns raised by the new frontier of human embryo stem cell research. Even the most noble ends do not justify any means.

My position on these issues is shaped by deeply held beliefs. I'm a strong supporter of science and technology, and believe they have the potential for incredible good—to improve lives, to save life, to conquer disease. Research offers hope that millions of our loved ones may be cured of a disease and rid of their suffering. I have friends whose chil-dren suffer from juvenile diabetes. Nancy Reagan has written me about President Reagan's struggle with Alzheimer's. My own family has con-fronted the tragedy of childhood leukemia. And, like all Americans, I have great hope for cures.

I also believe human life is a sacred gift from our Creator. I worry about a culture that devalues life, and believe as your President I have an important obligation to foster and encourage respect for life in America and throughout the world. And while we're all hopeful about the potential of this research, no one can be certain that the science will live up to the hope it has generated.

Eight years ago, scientists believed fetal tissue research offered great hope for cures and treatments—yet, the progress to date has not lived up to its initial expectations. Embryonic stem cell research offers both great promise and great peril. So I have decided we must proceed with great care.

As a result of private research, more than 60 genetically diverse stem cell lines already exist. They were created from embryos that have already been destroyed, and they have the ability to regenerate themselves indefinitely, creating ongoing opportunities for research. I have concluded that we should allow federal funds to be used for research on these existing stem cell lines, where the life and death decision has already been made.

Leading scientists tell me research on these 60 lines has great promise that could lead to breakthrough therapies and cures. This allows us to explore the promise and potential of stem cell research without crossing a fundamental moral line, by providing taxpayer funding that would sanction or encourage further destruction of human embryos that have at least the potential for life.

I also believe that great scientific progress can be made through aggressive federal funding of research on umbilical cord, placenta, adult, and animal stem cells which do not involve the same moral dilemma. This year, your government will spend $250 million on this important research.

I will also name a President's council to monitor stem cell research, to recommend appropriate guidelines and regulations, and to consider all of the medical and ethical ramifications of biomedical innovation. This council will consist of leading scientists, doctors, ethicists, lawyers, theologians and others, and will be chaired by Dr. Leon Kass, a leading biomedical ethicist from the University of Chicago.

This council will keep us apprised of new developments and give our nation a forum to continue to discuss and evaluate these important issues. As we go forward, I hope we will always be guided by both intellect and heart, by both our capabilities and our conscience.

I have made this decision with great care, and I pray it is the right one.

Thank you for listening. Good night, and God bless America.

END 8:12 P.M. CDT

APPENDIX ITEM II: BACKGROUNDER ON STEM CELL RESEARCH FROM THE NATIONAL INSTITUTES OF HEALTH

The following information on stem cells and stem cell research from the National Institutes of Health (NIH) provides a good summary of the current state of stem cell research and supplies a brief summary of the restrictions placed by President George W. Bush on the federal funding for embryonic stem cell research.

NIH Backgrounder on Stem Cells

What are Stem Cells?

Stem cells have the remarkable potential to develop into many different cell types in the body. Serving as a sort of repair system for the body, they can theoretically divide without limit to replenish other cells as long as the person or animal is still alive. When a stem cell divides, each new cell has the potential to either remain a stem cell or become another type of cell with a more specialized function, such as a muscle cell, a red blood cell, or a brain cell.

What Classes of Stem Cells are There?

Common terms you may come across describing stem cells group them according to how many different types of cells they have the potential to produce. A fertilized egg is considered **totipotent**, meaning that its potential is total; it gives rise to all the different types of cells in the body. **Pluripotent** stem cells can give rise to any type of cell in the body except those needed to develop a fetus. Stem cells that can give rise to multiple different cell types are generally called **multipotent**.

Why are Doctors and Scientists so Excited About Stem Cells?

Stem cells have potential in many different areas of health and medical research. To start with, studying stem cells will help us to understand how they transform into the dazzling array of specialized cells that make us what we are. Some of the most serious medical conditions, such as cancer and birth defects, are due to problems that occur somewhere in this process. A better understanding of normal cell development will allow us to understand and perhaps correct the errors that cause these medical conditions.

Another potential application of stem cells is making cells and tissues for medical therapies. Today, donated organs and tissues are often used to replace those that are diseased or destroyed. Unfortunately, the number of people suffering from these disorders far outstrips the number of organs available for transplantation. Stem cells offer the possibility of a renewable source of replacement cells and tissues to treat myriad diseases, conditions, and disabilities including Parkinson's and Alzheimer's diseases, spinal cord injury, stroke, burns, heart disease, diabetes, osteoarthritis, and rheumatoid arthritis. There is almost no realm of medicine that might not be touched by this innovation.

Have Stem Cells Been Used Successfully to Treat any Human Diseases Yet?

Blood-forming stem cells in bone marrow called hematopoietic stem cells (HSCs) are currently the only type of stem cell commonly used for therapy. Doctors have been transferring HSCs in bone marrow transplants for over 40 years. More advanced techniques of collecting, or "harvesting," HSCs are now used in order to treat leukemia, lymphoma, and several inherited blood disorders.

The clinical potential of stem cells has also been demonstrated in the treatment of other human diseases that include diabetes and advanced kidney cancer. However, these newer applications have involved studies with a very limited number of patients, using stem cells that were harvested from people.

How do Scientists Get Stem Cells for Medical and Scientific Use?

Pluripotent stem cells have been isolated from human embryos that are a few days old. Cells from these embryos can be used to create pluripotent stem cell "lines," cultures that can be grown indefinitely in the laboratory. Multipotent stem cell lines have also been developed from fetal tissue obtained from terminated pregnancies.

Stem cells can also be isolated from adult tissue. Thus far, these cells have been multipotent. Adult stem cells have not been found for all types of tissue, but discoveries in this area of research are increasing. For example, until recently it was thought that stem cells were not present in the adult nervous system, but in recent years such stem cells have been found in the brain.

Why do Scientists Want to Use Stem Cell Lines?

Once a stem cell line is established from a cell in the body, it is essentially immortal, no matter how it was derived. That is, it does not have to be created again from the original embryo or adult. Once established, it can be grown in the laboratory indefinitely and widely distributed to other researchers.

In addition, before scientists can use any type of stem cell for transplantation, they must overcome attempts by a patient's immune system to reject the transplant. Human stem cell lines might in the future be modified with gene therapy or other techniques to overcome this immune rejection. Scientists might also be able to replace damaged genes or add new genes to stem cells in order to give them new characteristics that can ultimately help to treat diseases.

What Will be the Best Type of Stem Cell to Use for Therapy?

Pluripotent stem cells, while having great therapeutic potential, face formidable technical challenges. First, scientists must learn how to control their development into all the different types of cells in the body. Second, the cells now available for research are likely to be rejected by a patient's immune system. Another serious consideration is that the idea of using stem cells from human embryos or human fetal tissue troubles many people on ethical grounds.

Until recently, there was little evidence that stem cells from adults could change course and provide the flexibility that researchers need in order to address all the medical diseases and disorders they would like to. New findings in animals, however, suggest that even after a stem cell has begun to specialize, it may be more flexible than previously thought.

There are currently several limitations to using adult stem cells. Although many different kinds of multipotent stem cells have been identified, the evidence that adult stem cells could give rise to all cell and tissue types is not yet conclusive. Adult stem cells are often present in only minute quantities and can therefore be difficult to isolate and purify. There is also evidence that they may not have the same capacity to multiply as embryonic stem cells do. Finally, adult stem cells may contain more DNA abnormalities—caused by sunlight, toxins and errors in making more DNA copies during the course of a lifetime. These potential weaknesses might limit the usefulness of adult stem cells.

Does NIH Fund Embryonic Stem Cell Research?

Research on human embryonic stem cell lines may receive NIH funding if the cell line meets the following criteria: removal of cells from the embryo must have been initiated before August 9, 2001, when President Bush outlined this policy; and the embryo from which the stem cell line was derived must no longer have had the possibility of developing further as a human being. The embryo must have been created for reproductive purposes but no longer be needed for them. Informed consent must have been obtained from the parent(s) for the donation of the embryo, and no financial inducements for donation are allowed.

In order to ensure that federal funds are used to support only stem cell research that is scientifically sound, legal, and ethical, NIH examines stem cell lines and maintains a registry of those lines that satisfy the criteria at http://stemcells.nih.gov/research/registry.

Which Research Is Best to Pursue?

The development of stem cell lines that can produce many tissues of the human body is an important scientific breakthrough. This research has the potential to revolutionize the practice of medicine and improve the quality and length of life. Given the enormous promise of stem cells therapies for so many devastating diseases, NIH believes that it is important to simultaneously pursue all lines of research and search for the very best sources of these cells.

A more detailed primer on stem cells can be found at http://stemcells.nih.gov/info/basics/. For current, in-depth information on NIH and stem cell research, visit http://stemcells.nih.gov/index.asp.

APPENDIX ITEM III: PREPARED REMARKS BY VICE ADMIRAL RICHARD H. CARMONA, M.D., M.P.H, FACS, UNITED STATES SURGEON GENERAL, ON ORGAN DONATION IN THE 21ST CENTURY AS THE BASIS OF HIS SPEECH BEFORE A MEETING OF THE JOINT COMMISSION ON ACCREDITATION OF HEALTHCARE ORGANIZATIONS, MARCH 10, 2004.

The lack of donor organs to meet the demand by critically ill patients is discussed in length in Chapters 2 and 5 and remains a primary stumbling block in the full use of transplantation to help patients suffering from end-stage organ failure. Over the years both the transplant community and government agencies have struggled with efforts to improve donation rates and close the gap between the need for organs and the availability of suitable organs for transplantation. In this speech, the surgeon general addresses this issue and discusses such efforts as the government's Gift of Life Donation Initiative and a public awareness and education campaign called Healthy Lifestyles & Disease Prevention. As a public health professional, the surgeon general emphasizes not only the importance of improving organ donation rates but also fundamental public health principles such as the need to increase awareness about healthy living to prevent diseases that lead to end-stage organ failure and discrepancies in the availability of health care depending largely on socioeconomic factors. This speech can also be accessed at the U.S. Department of Health & Human Services Web site at http://www.surgeongeneral.gov/news/speeches/JCAHOOrgan_03102004.htm.

Remarks as prepared; not a transcript
Vice Admiral Richard H. Carmona, M.D., M.P.H, FACS
United States Surgeon General
U.S. Department of Health and Human Services
Joint Commission on Accreditation of Healthcare Organizations
Wednesday, March 10, 2004
Washington, D.C.

"Organ Donation in the 21st Century: National Efforts to Narrow the Gap"

Thank you, Dennis (Dennis O'Leary, M.D., JCAHO President), for that terrific introduction.

It's great to be here with all of you today.

Today's topic: closing the gap between the more than 83,000 people who need an organ to save or enhance their lives, and the donations needed from fellow citizens and family members who can give the Gift of Life, is one that is very important to me and to my boss, Secretary Thompson.

My official title may be Surgeon General, but one of my most important titles is "Organ Donor," . . . and my family knows about it!

I have seen this issue from a very basic level.

As a trauma surgeon in an emergency room, I watched when family members facing the most difficult crisis of their lives—the loss of a child or spouse—also wrestled with the difficult decision of whether or not to donate that child or spouse's organs and tissues.

Those of you who have been through it yourselves know that it is both heartbreaking and life-giving at the same time. Families devastated by the loss of a loved one can take comfort in knowing that their loved one's organs and tissues have saved or improved up to 50 other lives.

And now, of course, I am seeing the issue from a new vantage point—that of Surgeon General.

I see the numbers—more than 83,000 people waiting for transplants, 18 of whom die each day.

Those numbers represent real people, with real lives, with loved ones who wait expectantly, and hopefully, and perhaps fearfully, knowing they cannot control the outcome but must depend on the good will of others.

I see the discrepancies between donation levels at various major hospitals.

I hear the myths surrounding the issue of organ donation, which prevent innumerable people from giving the Gift of Life.

And like Secretary Thompson, whose very first initiative as leader of Health and Human Services was to implement the *Gift of Life Donation Initiative*, I want to work hard to close the gap.

When President Bush and Secretary Thompson nominated me to be Surgeon General, they asked me to focus on three priorities to maintain and improve the health of the American people.

All three of my priorities are evidence-based. They are: prevention, public health preparedness, and eliminating health care disparities. Woven through all these issues that constitute my portfolio is health literacy. Today I will speak about health literacy and the relationship of all these priorities to organ donation.

Prevention

Seven of 10 Americans who die each year die of a chronic disease. Most of these diseases are preventable by relatively simple steps: healthy eating, being active and making healthy choices, such as not smoking and avoiding alcohol and drugs.

There is no greater imperative in American health care than switching from a treatment-oriented society, to a prevention-oriented society.

Right now we've got it backwards. We wait years and years, doing nothing about unhealthy eating habits and lack of physical activity, or poor choices about smoking, alcohol, and drugs, until people get sick.

Then we spend lots of money on costly treatments to make them well, often when it is already too late.

The paradox of modern health care is this: while medical technology is pushing forward at a breathtaking rate, helping us to save more lives than ever, our behavior as individuals has not kept pace.

In 1954, surgeons removed a kidney from one identical twin and placed it in the other. That was the first organ transplant. Just 50 years ago. In 2002, almost 25,000 transplants were performed. Organ transplantation is truly a miracle of modern medicine.

But as our ability to perform these operations more successfully grows, so does the *need* for them, as illnesses leading to organ failure, such as diabetes and high blood pressure, continue to increase.

Tobacco-related illness kills 435,000 American a year. Obesity-related illness is catching up quickly, now resulting in 400,000 deaths each year.

Yesterday the Secretary announced an innovative public awareness and education campaign called *Healthy Lifestyles & Disease Prevention.*

The campaign encourages American families to take *small, manageable steps* within their current lifestyle—versus drastic changes—to ensure effective, long-term weight control.

Also, NIH is developing a Strategic Plan for Obesity Research which will explore prevention and treatment approaches that encompass behavioral, socio-cultural, environmental, and genetic factors contributing to obesity.

As we bring about change in the lifestyles and choices of Americans—a long, difficult process to be sure—we will very gradually reduce the need for organ donation.

Public Health Preparedness

My second priority is public health preparedness.

We are investing the resources at the federal, state, and local levels to strengthen the public health system and to prevent, mitigate, and respond to all-hazards emergencies.

As we prepare for emergencies by funding hospitals, state and local trauma and EMS systems, and other partners, we are also building a stronger public health system.

And we are better prepared to meet traditional public health needs, such as emerging illness and immunization.

Eliminating Health Care Disparities

My third priority is working to eliminate health care disparities.

The scientific evidence is crystal clear: Many individuals from minority communities suffer a greater burden of death and disease from breast cancer, prostate cancer, cervical cancer, cardiovascular disease, and other illnesses.

At HHS we are working hard to eliminate health disparities through our research institutes, such as the National Center on Minority Health and Health Disparities and the National Cancer Institute and our outreach efforts such as *Take a Loved One to the Doctor Day.*

And the President has kept his commitment to expand Community Health Centers to serve more people, many in communities of color.

In the last three years, we have expanded access for an additional 3 million people through 614 new and expanded sites.

We need to do more to eliminate disparities, which are also present when it comes to organ donation. Finding a matching donor is much easier when the patient and donor share a similar heritage or ethnicity.

While minorities have typically donated in proportion to their percentages of the population, they have a higher need for transplants due to the higher incidence of disease they face.

Health Literacy

There's a widespread problem slowing down our progress in all three of these public health priority areas, and it's directly related to 'closing the gap' in organ donation.

The problem is *low* health literacy. Health literacy is the ability of an individual to access, understand, and use health-related information and services to make appropriate health decisions.

Consider this: A recent study of English-speaking patients in public hospitals revealed that one-third were unable to read basic health materials. 26 percent of the patients could not read their appointment slips, and 42 percent did not understand the labels on their prescription bottles.

Further studies show that people of all ages, races, incomes, and education levels are challenged by *low* health literacy.

Not every American is a scientist or a health care professional, and we can't expect everyone to understand what it takes health care professionals years of training to learn.

National efforts to increase public awareness and donations

Perhaps nowhere in medicine is the need for improved health literacy more pronounced than in organ donation.

Many Americans simply do not know the facts about organ donation.

And as we know, in the absence of good information, bad information thrives.

The myths out there about organ donation range from the "seemingly logical"—"I have a history of illness; you wouldn't want my organs"—to the absurd, "If the hospital knows I am a donor, they will not try to save my life if I am in an accident."

How do we overcome those myths? Better information.

And better information will lead to increased donation. According to a 2001 study by the Agency for Healthcare Research and Quality (AHRQ), organ donations increase when families have good information about the donation process.

The study found that:

*Families who knew about a patient's wishes were seven times more likely to donate organs than families who were unsure; and

*Families who met with organ donation professionals about the donation process were more than three times likely to donate organs than families who did not.

So Secretary Thompson has made increasing public awareness and promoting organ, tissue, marrow, and blood donation the heart of his *Gift of Life Donation Campaign*.

His goal is to reach all Americans through:

*The Workplace Partnership for Life. Nearly 10,000 companies and organizations have signed up and have committed to build donor awareness among their employees;

*A model organ donor card—so donors can easily share their decision to be donors with loved ones and co-workers;

*A model donation education package for high schools and driver's education programs—so our nation's youth will be prepared to make the donation decision that is right for them when they obtain their first driver's license;

*A national forum on organ donor registries, which looks at ways to improve the system.

We are also working to increase public awareness through the media. Last fall, the HHS-funded PBS documentary "No Greater Love," which highlighted the critical need for donors, won an Emmy.

We have done special media targeting in minority communities—$2 million in the last year in radio ads and printed materials in 15 media markets with the highest numbers of Hispanics and African Americans.

These are only some of the ways we are working to "get the word out"—to improve health literacy—about organ donation. Many of you here today also are engaged in a myriad of activities to promote donation in communities, schools, hospitals and other venues.

And it is working. Secretary Thompson announced last month that organ donation is up 4.8 percent for the first 11 months of 2003.

This is the most significant organ donation increase since 1998.

There is also very promising news when it comes to minorities: in 2003, donations among Hispanics increased by nearly 14%, and donations among African-Americans increased by more than 11%.

National efforts to increase donation through the Secretary's Organ Donation Breakthrough Collaborative

In addition to increasing public awareness and making it easier for people to make and share their decision to become donors, we are also working with hospitals and Organ Procurement Organizations to generate increases in organ donation.

Most hospitals have donation rates ranging from 30 [to] 55% of their potential donors.

Some hospitals, though, have donation rates over 75%, so clearly there are discrepancies in the way the donation process works in various hospitals. We are working to "close this gap" as well.

Last fall Secretary Thompson joined leaders of large hospitals and organ procurement organizations to release a study profiling the practices being used by these successful organizations to achieve high organ donation rates.

At the same time, leaders from other hospitals spent two days learning about these "best practices" and returned to their institutions to design and implement changes to increase donation rates.

We are pleased with the progress of the Secretary's *Organ Donation Breakthrough Collaborative*, and the support the Join Commission has shown for this initiative.

Charge

HHS is working in many ways to "close the gap" between the more than 83,000 people who need organs and the donors who can give them. But we must all work together in partnership: government, medical systems, doctors, Organ Procurement Organizations, employers, and families to make our vision of "No Greater Love" a reality.

Greater love has no one than this, than to lay down one's life for his friends (John 15:13).

Americans are the most generous people on earth, and my belief is that when they know the facts about organ donation, and when we provide them the means to indicate their wishes in a simple way, they will respond overwhelmingly in their willingness to give the gift of life to others if their own lives are cut tragically short.

Let's keep working together on this most noble cause. Thank you.

APPENDIX ITEM IV: SELECTION OF SUMMARY MEETING NOTES ABOUT AMENDING THE NATIONAL ORGAN TRANSPLANT ACT (NOTA) GIVEN AT A MEETING OF THE U.S. DEPARTMENT OF HEALTH AND HUMAN SERVICES ADVISORY COMMITTEE ON ORGAN TRANSPLANTATION, NOVEMBER 4–5, 2004.

The following summary focuses on two issues concerned with increasing the supply of donor organs. It reflects concerns and various considerations over ethical issues associated with transplantation, such as the sale of organs, black markets, and maintaining an individual's autonomy over his or her own body.

The first part of the summary focuses on "valuable consideration," which, in legal terms, is part of a contract that confers benefit on the other party, in this case, organ donors. Valuable considerations typically encompass money, work, performance, assets, or some other type of benefit given to the other party for a service or duty performed. The following discussion seeks to establish what are fair and legitimate practices that offer benefits to organ donors while ensuring that a commercial market is not created in which organs are bought and sold.

The second part of the proposed amendment deals with the idea of presumed consent, that is, that organs can be automatically harvested from people who die if there is no record of the patient objecting to the process or objections from family members or others who are legally sanctioned to make decisions for the individual. Here the focus is on encouraging federal sponsorships of state initiatives to study making organ donations under a presumed consent plan.

The entire summary meeting notes for the November 2004 meeting of the Advisory Committee on Organ Transplantation can be found at http://www.organdonor.gov/acot11-2004.htm.

Advisory Committee on Organ Transplantation
November 4–5, 2004
Doubletree Hotel and Executive Meeting
Rockville, Maryland
Thursday November 4, 2004

Proposal to Amend Section 301 of the National Organ Transplant Act (NOTA)

Gail Agrawal

The Valuable Consideration Subcommittee (Subcommittee A) presented recommendations related to two issues: valuable consideration and presumed consent.

Valuable Consideration

Ms. Agrawal recalled discussions at the May ACOT meeting about why it would be desirable to get clarification and greater specificity in regard to the broad and somewhat confusing prohibition of valuable consideration in the context of organ donation. This subcommittee proposed that the Secretary seek some authority to define the prohibition on valuable consideration through amendment of existing regulations to provide for beneficial and ethical means to promote organ donation.

Ms. Agrawal drafted some language for a recommendation, which has been reviewed by HRSA staff:

The Advisory Committee on Organ Transplantation (ACOT) recommends that the Secretary of Health and Human Services seek authority to identify and exclude certain practices from the definition of "valuable consideration" in section 301(a) of the National Organ Transplant Act, as amended. The Secretary's authority should be limited to legitimate and beneficial practices that are intended to increase the supply of human organs, without creating a commercial market for the purchase or sale of human organs or posing a risk of coercion of a potential donor or donor family. In addition, the Secretary should be required to obtain an appropriate independent ethical evaluation before excluding any practice from the prohibition on valuable consideration.

ACOT has concluded that a process to limit the scope of "valuable consideration" would encourage the development of ethical practices to increase the supply of human organs and provide certainty to the transplant community about the scope of permissible activities. Regulatory authority is both more flexible and more responsive to innovation than an expanded statutory list of practices that are not included in the term "valuable consideration." The notice and comment period will provide an opportunity for public and professional input into any proposed regulation.

ACOT, therefore, recommends that Section 301 of the National Organ Transplant Act be amended in its entirety to read as follows:

(a) Prohibition

It shall be unlawful for any person to knowingly acquire, receive, or otherwise transfer any human organ for valuable consideration for use in human transplantation if the transfer affects interstate commerce.

(b) Penalties

Any person who violates subsection (a) of this section shall be fined not more than $50,000 or imprisoned not more than five years, or both.

(c) Definitions

For purposes of subsection (a) of this section:

(1) The term "human organ" means the human (including fetal) kidney, liver, heart, lung, pancreas, bone marrow, cornea, eye, bone, and skin or any subpart thereof and any other human organ (or any subpart thereof, including that derived from a fetus) specified by the Secretary of Health and Human Services by regulation.

(2) The term "valuable consideration" does not include the reasonable payments associated with the removal, transportation, implantation, processing, preservation, quality control, and storage of a human organ, the expenses of travel, housing, and lost wages incurred by the donor of a human organ in connection with the donation of the organ, *or such other practices that the Secretary of Health and Human Services shall designate by regulation pursuant to subsection (d) of this section.*

(3) The term "interstate commerce" has the meaning prescribed for it by section 321(b) of Title 21.

(d) The Secretary of Health and Human Services shall propose and promulgate regulations to ensure that interpretations of subsection (c)(2) do not impede legitimate and beneficial practices that are intended to increase the supply of human organs available for transplantation, provided, however, that any practice that poses a risk of coercion in connection with the donation of a human organ or of the creation of a commercial market for the purchase or sale of human organs is not a legitimate or beneficial practice within the meaning of this subsection (d). In considering legitimate and beneficial practices that will be excluded from the prohibition on valuable consideration set forth in subsection (c)(2), the Secretary shall seek an ethical evaluation from an appropriate entity, including without limitation the Institute of Medicine and the President's Council on Bioethics, or such similar or successor entity."

Ms. Agrawal observed that this approach would preclude the creation of a commercial market and it cannot enrich donors. We do not want the rewards to be so great as to generate a coercive effect. We also provided a mechanism for an ethical review of the proposal prior to being put out for the notice and comment period. The effect of this recommendation is to bring the idea of clarifying valuable consideration to the fore. Ultimately, congressional action would be required.

Frank Delmonico applauded this effort because ACOT would be opposing commercial markets in organs for transplantation. Hans Sollinger commented that the recent Denver case plus the fact that some 500,000 people are on dialysis indicate that this measure may not be enough. He commented that a presentation by Janet Radcliffe-Richards in Vienna intrigued him about the idea of having a controlled system operating above the table to monitor what happens. He said that the growing demand for organs in the coming years will likely drive a black market in organs: "We must offer oversight; we cannot just say, don't do it." Dr. Ascher advocated oversight without commercialization. Ms. Agrawal said that the recommendation reflects the opinion of the subcommittee—purchase and sale of organs are not permissible. If we want to consider purchase and sale, then the subcommittee does not want to offer this recommendation.

Bill Harmon asked if this proposed amendment of NOTA would preclude the Wisconsin tax benefit. Ms. Agrawal responded that the Secretary and HHS staff would have to make that determination. In her opinion, that would not be purchase or sale of an organ. Whether it constitutes coercion or purchase/sale would be a question to address. Emily Marcus Levine observed that the Wisconsin law is permissible because it reimburses for donor expenses already allowable under NOTA.

There was some discussion about whether OPOs can help people find matching donors outside the construct of for-profit organizations. The concept of someone being monetarily enriched by donating organs is the problematic area. We need to find an ethical way to bring people together.

Dr. Sollinger said that presently some altruistic individuals are becoming living donors, but the situation is likely to move away from an altruistic approach and to move toward commercial markets in organs, such as those that exist in Pakistan and India. ACOT has heard only one side of this issue and the world does not necessarily agree with the view we are trying to support. Dr. Sollinger suggested that ACOT should invite speakers to present the other side. Several participants suggested moving forward on this recommendation because ACOT has been opposed to pure buying and selling of organs. Nevertheless, ACOT should consider hearing from presenters on the more controversial topic of commercial markets in organs. Dr. Harmon said that this recommendation would allow us to go forward. If we open the question about buying and selling organs today, we will not be able to reach an agreement soon. This step does not prohibit the next step. He noted that some nations (e.g., Kuwait) have reconsidered and eliminated their buy/sell market.

Carlton Young pointed out that we have a limited resource that we are trying to parcel out. We are trying to protect the disenfranchised while trying to implement everything we can do improve organ donation. We must improve the supply side.

Dr. Ascher then moved to insert the word "unregulated" before the word "commercial." Dr. Sollinger seconded the motion. Ms. Agrawal called for further discussion. Ms. Agrawal cautioned that such a modification of the proposal might imply the obverse of the statement's intent. Dr. Delmonico said that if we open the door for a regulated market, then we will be going back to ground zero. Dr. Ascher responded that we do not know where this field is going. Adding the word "unregulated" gives us some modicum of control. Dr. Harmon said he agreed with Dr. Delmonico, that this recommendation will be a lightning rod if accepted. Ms. Turrisi suggested taking out the word "commercial." The word "unregulated" is important. Ms. Solarz said that substituting this language is likely intended to give us flexibility down the road because it takes so much time to get a regulation through the process. Nevertheless, this is a slippery slope. Those who are disenfranchised by our health care system would be exploited. It would be anathema to allow people to sell pieces of themselves, even in a regulated situation. She said she would not back this proposed modification. It pains her to think that our system could encourage selling of organs even if regulated. We must be above that. We have an organ shortage, but we cannot have people risk themselves because they do not have what they need.

Dr. Sollinger said that it is not necessarily true that the poor and disadvantaged will bear the brunt of this (buying/selling of organs). But, that does happen every day. Think of how many of the rich and famous are serving in Iraq. He expressed concern that we are facing an eventual black market in organs. It has happened already in so-called civilized countries. We must be realistic. We have been very unilateral, but we must expand this discussion.

Amadeo Marcos stated that it is the transplant center that has the ultimate control in preventing black markets. Dr. Delmonico said that the American Society for Transplantation has discussed a commercial market in organs, but has expressed its opposition. The Congress considered it via Senator Frist's bill and rejected it. It was rejected by Senator Kennedy's staff as well. Just because a black market might be coming is no justification for creating a regulated market in organs, according to Dr. Delmonico. Ms. Agrawal called a vote to amend the language in the proposed recommendation by inserting the word "unregulated" before the word "commercial." The vote was 4 for, 9 opposed, 2 abstentions. The motion failed.

Ms. Agrawal called a vote to adopt the recommendation as originally written (and reproduced above). The vote was 15 for, 0 opposed, 1 abstention. The motion passed, and the recommendation was adopted as written.

Presumed Consent

Ms. Agrawal recalled that Phil Berry has previously presented to ACOT on the topic of presumed consent. Moving toward a presumed consent model would have to be done at the State level because the Uniform Anatomical Gift Act (UAGA), which make provisions for consent is a State law, not a Federal law. The subcommittee proposes language for a recommendation to encourage the Secretary to support State initiatives for demonstration or pilot projects for making anatomical gifts under a presumed consent model:

The Advisory Committee on Organ Transplantation (ACOT) recommends that the Secretary of Health and Human Services encourage States to undertake demonstration projects to test the feasibility of adopting a model of presumed consent to organ donation. The current system for the donation of human organs from deceased donors is based on a default assumption that individuals prefer not to donate their organs after their death. A policy of presumed consent would include as a default assumption that individuals do prefer to donate their organs for transplantation at death. Because of the life-saving potential of transplantation, a presumed consent model would be a moral improvement over the current system, provided individual autonomy is appropriately protected through a system of declining to donate.

The Advisory Committee on Organ Transplantation, therefore, recommends that the Secretary authorize, encourage, and support State demonstration projects to design and implement "presumed consent" models for making anatomical gifts. The precise design of such models should be left to the states, provided that any State demonstration project authorized by the Secretary shall include provisions to ensure adequate notification and education of the citizens of the State and a method designed to permit any person not wishing to consent to an anatomical gift at death to register a decision to refuse to make an anatomical gift.

Ms. Agrawal envisions that a State could come to HHS with a proposal and bring the design to the Secretary with parameters and safeguards. The Secretary and staff would review the proposal. The object would be to see if these programs might increase the supply of organs.

Dr. Berry moved to approve the recommendation. Dr. Delmonico seconded the motion. Ms. Agrawal opened the floor for further discussion.

Susan Gunderson moved to change the words "consent to an anatomical gift" in the last sentence to "authorize an anatomical gift." Dr. Berry seconded the motion. Ms. Agrawal asked for discussion. She said that under a presumed consent model it is different from an anatomical gift. The default position is non-authorization. Mr. Seely warned that the phrase "presumed consent" has been used for years now. We do not want to muddy the waters or distract from the important issue at hand. Ms. Gunderson suggested changing only the last sentence and not the title of the recommendation.

Mike Seely said that States that have registries in place might be able to see if a presumed consent model would affect donation rates. Dr. Berry mentioned that he celebrated his 18th birthday last week (18 years since his liver transplant). More than 87,000 people are on the waitlist for livers now. We must look at alternatives. It is speculated that presumed consent or presumed authorization might be better, but it is mere speculation until we do it. Any State that has the wherewithal to make it happen should be allowed to do so for several years to be an adequate test to see once and for all whether it makes a difference. If a handful of States undertake such demonstrations and show a positive change in donation rates, then we can say that presumed consent is a viable alternative to what we are doing now. Until we do the studies, we will keep talking about it. It is time to see if it will work.

Ms. Agrawal called for a vote on proposing the recommendation with the following change: In the last sentence, change the words "consent to an anatomical gift" in to "authorize an anatomical gift." The vote was 14 for, 0 opposed, 0 abstentions. The motion passed, and the recommendation was adopted as amended.

APPENDIX ITEM V: SELECTION OF SUMMARY MEETING NOTES ABOUT LIVING DONORS AND OPTN ORGAN-ALLOCATION PLANS GIVEN AT A MEETING OF THE U.S. DEPARTMENT OF HEALTH AND HUMAN SERVICES ADVISORY COMMITTEE ON ORGAN TRANSPLANTATION, NOVEMBER 1, 2005.

Live organ donors represent an increasingly important avenue for obtaining much needed organs to save lives. As discussed in Chapter 8, there are several ethical considerations surrounding the use of perfectly healthy individuals to obtain organs. Although the operation that live kidney and liver donors undergo to provide part of their organs is relatively safe, risks are involved and abuses can occur. In the following segments taken from the 2005 summary report of an Advisory Committee on Organ Transplantation meeting, a living donor registry is discussed. Such a registry is needed in the view of many to determine the long-term health outcomes, both physical and mental, for people who are living donors.

The second segment taken from the summary report is about OPTN's efforts to improve organ allocation policies, including the oversight of live organ donations.

The entire report summary of this meeting can be obtained online at http://www.organdonor.gov/acot11-2005.htm.

Advisory Committee on Organ Transplantation (ACOT)
Fall Meeting
November 1, 2005
Convened by Conference Call
Report on Issues in Developing a Living Donor Registry
Jim Burdick, M.D., Director, Division of Transplantation

Only in recent years has HHS been involved in a major way with living donations. There has been an explosion of opportunities in the area of living donors.

The OPTN is tasked with getting information on every living donor of an organ after 1 and 2 years of donation. HHS has funded a study of young living donors through adulthood. There are NIH studies that are predominantly physiological, hypothesis-driven scientific investigations of living donors. These provide a check and balance of health outcomes and patient safety.

Right now the ACOT is in a position to direct the desired content of the living donor registry. Dr. Burdick asked the members what they would like to see in terms of follow-up efforts with living donors. Should donors be surveyed every year for the rest of their lives, or would that be too cumbersome? After the first two years, should contact be done at 5, 10, and 15 years out? What would be the role and services provided by a hotline for donors? Should subsistence expenses be covered for disadvantaged donors?

One area not well served is the examination of the psychological/mental health impact on living donors.

Dr. Burdick also noted that there is disturbing evidence that some sites may not be applying effective screening of potential donors (e.g., there are instances of kidney donors having renal failure themselves within 5 years of donation). An emphasis on renal failure protection needs to be applied. Dr. Roger Evans noted that there is a need to know if past donors who are on the waiting list themselves were higher risk to begin with, or if there were other factors introduced after donation.

Kathy Turrisi stated that there are more living donors than ever before—this increase could be accounted for partially by decreased selectivity for living donors. There seem anecdotally to be more problems with donors than in the past; diligent follow up to assess what is going on is needed to be transparent as a community.

Rhonda Boone noted that 1- and 2-year follow-up is a good start, but not good enough. More long-term follow-up is needed. Additionally, there are quality of life issues that potential donors need to be informed about.

Dr. Burdick stated that various programs have studied kidney donors 10-15 years after donation; but selection criteria are changing and might change validity of some of these studies. The OPTN is requiring 1- and 2-year reporting covering mortality and other medical data. Compliance with this is not yet complete.

Ms. Boone noted that a tremendous number of liver donors have complications. Additionally, other quality of life issues, including lack of insurance, depression, divorce, and medical complications, need to be considered.

Roger Evans stated that there are other factors aside from donation that affect quality of life, and this needs to be kept in mind.

There is currently wide variation of criteria on who can be a donor. Ms. Turrisi suggested that more diligence is needed to protect donors. Dr. Burdick noted that there are guidelines for acceptance, but there are not mandates. One option is to specifically determine what constitutes due diligence.

Ms. Turrisi suggested collecting data and then subsequently eliminating the disincentive of out-of-pocket expenses of the donor.

Setting up a resource center for donors could be a cost-effective way to reach out to donors who feel isolated from their transplant center.

[Also included in summary meeting notes]

OPTN Strategic Plan for Organ Allocation
Frank Delmonico, M.D.,
President, United Network for Organ Sharing

Frank Delmonico thanked the ACOT for allowing him to make a presentation. The OPTN is implementing a strategic plan with five essential aspects:

• Increasing number of transplants and reducing wastage;
• The oversight of live organ donation and transplantation;
• The use of net benefit in the allocation of organs;
• Improving the efficiency, effectiveness, and equity of the OPTN's policies and processes.
• The collection of data targeted to the following goals: 1) assessment of performance; 2) development of policy; and 3) distribution of organs. Improving information technology and validating data.

In defining the strategic plan, OPTN called on a wide representation across the transplantation community to bring consensus and endorsement of the issues. As such, the plan is integrated with, and suggests courses of action and partnership opportunities for, other key stakeholders in the transplant community. Ways to assess progress are being developed and implemented, hard goals and targets have been established, collaboration is occurring to get the job done, and improvements and best practices are being identified and spread.

The first area of the strategic plan addresses methods to maximize the transplants performed from viable donor organs (reducing wastage). This includes changing perceptions of the use of DCD and ECD organs—e.g., for kidney transplants, these organs should be analyzed compared to ongoing dialysis rather than compared to ideal candidate organs. Another aspect of this issue is to standardize how a person is characterized as sensitized in tissue typing. Virtual crossmatching could take place, leading to:

• Decreased number of patients needing actual final crossmatch (No regional screen trays);

• Decreased time required for final crossmatching;

• Minimized wasted time crossmatching highly sensitized patients with known incompatibilities;

• Decreased CIT in some regions;

• Accelerated organ placement.

The second part of the strategic plan covers the oversight of live organ donation. The OPTN must have an emphasis on live donor safety. There is much interest in a live donor registry. The national organizations are concerned about the health of the donor. If there's a peri-operative death of donor, it should get reported to the OPTN Membership and Professional Standards Committee as an event. If a live donor is in need of a transplant in the peri-operative period, it should get reported to the OPTN Membership and Professional Standards Committee as an event.

Concern for the protection and well-being of the living donor prompted the transplant community to develop a Consensus Statement on the Live Organ Donor:

• The person who gives consent to be a live organ donor should be competent, willing to donate, free of coercion, medically and psychosocially suitable, fully informed of the risks and benefits as a donor, and fully informed of risks, benefits, and alternative treatment available to recipient.

• The benefits to both donor and recipient must outweigh the risks associated with the donation and transplantation of the living donor organ. Donors should not be called upon to donate in clinically hopeless situations. [JAMA 2000; 284: 2919 – 2926]

Dr. Delmonico took questions:

One ACOT member asked what is being done to look at kidney donors who have themselves ended up on the waiting list?

Dr. Delmonico stated that there have been inquiries as to why this is occurring; the individuals themselves get priority on the waiting list.

Another member asked if there is an attempt to look at risk factors for these cases.

Dr. Delmonico stated that predilection to renal failure in the future should be screened, and that's a part of the inquiries.

Ms. Turrisi expressed concern that there are groups that are taking patients with morbidities. One ACOT member asked that quarterly report cards be provided on the areas of the OPTN strategic plan.

Dr. Delmonico stated that each of the work groups (each handling a different focus area) will be reporting. There will be a report in March, an assessment of progress with all of these items on the strategic plan.

APPENDIX ITEM VI: TRANSPLANTATION MYTHS

Many of the ethical concerns about transplantation, such as its high cost, the organ-donor shortage, and favoritism in the allocation of organs, have led to rumors, myths, and misunderstandings about transplantation. Myths about transplantation can be particularly dangerous because they may influence people in their decisions about whether or not to become an organ donor.

Although often myths and "urban legends" come from unofficial sources and are largely "stories" that have gained widespread attention by word of mouth or through the Internet, often the tabloid media will propagate these myths, as related in the following comprehensive story which appears on the United States Information Agency Web site at http://usinfo.state.gov/. It tells about the belief held by many residents in poorer countries in Latin America and other parts of the world that people have adopted or stolen babies to use them for their body parts. Also included in this appendix are the top ten myths concerning transplantation as listed by the Organ Procurement and Transplantation Network.

THE "BABY PARTS" MYTH: THE ANATOMY OF A RUMOR, UNITED STATES INFORMATION AGENCY, MAY 1996

Since 1987, a totally unfounded, horrifying rumor has swept the world press. The ghastly and totally untrue charge is that Americans—or Europeans, Canadians, or Israelis—are adopting infants or kidnapping children from Latin America or other locations, and murdering or maiming them in order to use their body parts for organ or cornea transplants. This gruesome story has been reported hundreds of times by newspapers, radio, and television stations throughout the world, has won prestigious journalism awards, and is believed by tens of millions of people, if not more.

The rumor turned deadly in Guatemala in 1994. On March 29, 1994, an American tourist, June Weinstock, was attacked by a mob who accused her of abducting a Guatemalan boy. Weinstock suffered multiple broken arms, internal injuries, and severe head injuries that have left her permanently incapacitated.

THE MYTHICAL ORIGINS OF THE RUMOR

The "baby parts" rumor probably arose spontaneously as an "urban legend," a false but widely believed form of modern folklore. There are many such widely repeated but totally unsubstantiated stories. For example, when microwave ovens began to be widely used, an apocryphal story began to circulate about a person who had tried to dry their wet dog in a microwave oven, only to have it explode. These word-of-mouth stories are typically said to have happened to "a friend of a friend," who can never be located because there is no factual basis for the rumor.

In the same way that fears about microwave technology led to this unfounded rumor, recent dramatic advances in organ transplantation have contributed to the "baby parts" myth. All of us may someday benefit from the gift of life that organ transplantation can provide. But the process also stirs powerful, primal anxieties. This was illustrated by the fictional 1978 American movie *Coma,* in which patients at a hospital were placed into comas so that corrupt doctors could "harvest" their organs for profit. The same fear of wrongful death and mutilation that formed the basis for this fictional thriller is at the root of the "baby parts" rumor.

Experts on popular myths state that the "baby parts" story is a modern adaptation of a centuries-old tale. French folklorist Veronique Campion-Vincent wrote:

"The baby-parts story is a new—updated and technologized—version of an immemorial fable. The core of the fable is that a group's children are being kidnapped and murdered by evil outsiders.

Accusations of such kidnappings and ritual murder were made against Christians in ancient Rome [and against] Jews throughout antiquity, the Middle Ages, and up to modern times. . . . Child abductions in 18th century France were explained by ailing nobility who needed them for medical reasons: the leprous King needed blood baths, or a mutilated Prince needed a new arm which incompetent surgeons were trying each day to graft from a new kidnapped child."

THE RUMOR BREAKS IN THE WORLD PRESS

In the modern version of this legend, individuals have reported hearing the "baby parts" rumor as far back as the early to mid-1980s, although it did not appear in the international press until January 1987, when Leonardo Villeda Bermudez, the former Secretary General of the Honduran Committee for Social Welfare, mentioned the rumor during an interview in a way that made it appear as if it was true. Mr. Villeda immediately issued a clarification stating that he had merely heard unconfirmed rumors of such activities. All top Honduran officials, including the President's wife, emphasized that there was no evidence for such allegations, but by this time the rumor had been reported by a wire service and it began to circulate throughout the media worldwide, appearing in Guatemala the next month and soon afterwards in Europe.

In April 1987, the Soviet disinformation apparatus began a conscious effort to spread and embellish this unfounded rumor. On April 5, 1987, Pravda carried the three-month-old Honduran story, citing the original allegations without mentioning subsequent press accounts dismissing the story. The Soviet news agency TASS replayed the story, and during 1987 and 1988 it appeared many times in the Soviet media and in pro-Soviet media worldwide. The Soviet disinformation campaign in the media ended in late 1988.

Occasional disinformation—deliberate lies or distortions undertaken for a political purpose—still occur. The Cubans continue to press the child organ trafficking story, having repeatedly tried to introduce resolutions on this issue at U.N. human rights meetings. One formerly Soviet-controlled front group, the International Association of Democratic Lawyers, has continued to try to foster the rumor, particularly through its status as a non-governmental organization accredited to the United Nations. Some anti-U.S. extremists, typically from the far left in Western Europe and the extreme right in Guatemala, have embraced the rumor enthusiastically, apparently because it fits with their anti-U.S. political agenda. Most recently, Iranian publications have begun to propagate the rumor.

Although political motivations have been responsible for some of the more spectacular outbursts of the child organ trafficking rumor, for the most part, the rumor has been embraced and spread by well-meaning individuals who believe it out of naivete or who worry that it may be true. Tragically, the publicity these well-intentioned individuals have given the rumor by deploring a non-existent crime has inadvertently contributed to its credibility and the resultant damage it has done. At this point, the rumor has attained such currency that it appears certain to continue on the strength of its own momentum for years to come.

THE IMPOSSIBILITY OF CONCEALING CLANDESTINE ORGAN TRANSPLANTS

Health and organ transplant officials in the United States and other countries have stated emphatically that it would be impossible to successfully conceal any clandestine organ trafficking ring.

In many countries, the sale or purchase of organs for transplants is expressly forbidden by law, with stiff penalties for violators. For example, organ sales for transplant have been illegal in the United States since 1984. There are similar statutes in many other countries.

In addition to the legal and moral deterrents to organ trafficking, the technical requirements that would be involved in arranging and operating an alleged murder-for-organ-transplantation scheme are so formidable that such clandestine activities are a practical impossibility.

In order for an organ transplantation to have any chance of success, a number of sophisticated medical procedures must be conducted to determine the suitability of various organs for transplantation and to permit a match with potential recipients. In particular, correct tissue and blood typing is critical to matching donor organs and potential transplant recipients. Crossing the blood group barrier from transplant donor to recipient can result in death. An equally important consideration is histocompatibility, which measures the extent to which a donor organ and a recipient match.

The surface of all cells in the body carries proteins known as major histocompatibility complex (MHC) antigens. These proteins act as signals that identify what is uniquely self to our immune system. The importance of matching MHC antigens for transplanted organs is similar to the need to match blood types for blood transfusions. However, MHC matches are more complex, and excessive differences between a donor and a recipient will cause the recipient's immune system to attack and reject the transplanted organ. In humans, the MHC antigens are encoded by a set of linked genes, which are designated as Human Leukocyte Antigens (HLA). In transplantation, it is vital to the survival and well-being of the recipient to identify and match the donor's HLA types. This can only be accomplished in a laboratory designed to test histocompatibility, and requires individuals with specialized laboratory skills to conduct the testing.

After the organs have been extracted from a donor, an extremely delicate and complex procedure that involves a transplant surgeon and support staff including an anesthesiologist, attending surgeons, and operating room nurses, the organs must be transported as rapidly as possible, typically by helicopter or airplane, to the hospitals where the transplants will occur. Before transporting the donor organ, special preservation solutions must be infused into it. Proper insulation and temperature controlled packaging including adequate ice or refrigeration must be used to protect the organ during shipment. Absolute sterile conditions must be maintained for the organ to remain viable for transplant.

Organ transplants must be accomplished extremely rapidly because the time that organs can survive outside the body is severely limited. Hearts must be transplanted within 5 hours, livers within 24 hours, pancreases within 6 to 12 hours, and lungs within 5 hours. Kidneys can survive the longest, but most surgeons will not transplant a kidney that was removed more than 48 hours before.

Sophisticated surgical equipment and highly skilled medical personnel are necessary for a transplant to take place. At a minimum, one needs 20 individuals, including three members of a surgical team, one scrub nurse, one circulating nurse, one anesthesiologist, one perfusion technician, and one general function technician. For all transplant surgery, a large area needed for the operating table, instrument table, laboratory instruments, anesthesia equipment, monitoring equipment, spare supplies, gas sources, and personnel access.

In addition, in order to prepare for a kidney recipient's surgery, a kidney machine must be available to perform dialysis. For a heart transplant, the patient must be placed on circulatory and respiratory bypass equipment during the entire length of the transplant procedure and constantly monitored by a pulmonary technologist. During a liver transplant, bleeding is extensive because the liver produces the substance that causes blood to coagulate. Access to a blood bank is necessary because as many as 20 to 50 units of blood may be required for blood transfusions.

Thus, the daunting technical requirements of the transplant process make it impossible that transplants could occur clandestinely, as the child organ trafficking rumor alleges. Such highly complex operations could not occur at hidden, makeshift facilities. It would not be possible to assemble a team of highly trained medical professionals who would all be willing to engage in such morally repugnant criminal acts and be willing to take the enormous personal risks that would be involved in performing a transplant operation clandestinely. Nor would it be possible to arrange such a procedure for purely logistical reasons alone because the technical resources required could not be assembled outside of major medical centers.

In addition, the transplant process does not end with the completion of the transplant operation. Follow-up care of the transplant recipient is critical for short-term and long-term survival and well-being. After the transplant operation, the organ recipient must be treated by a transplant physician, a separate individual from the transplant surgeon, who monitors, medicates, and treats the transplant recipient for the rest of his life. No transplant physician would treat a person without knowing all the circumstances of their progressive organ disease, the details of their transplant operation, including the identity and health records of the donor of the organ, and a great deal of other information that would not be available if the transplant operation were performed clandestinely.

It is important to remember that transplant surgeons and physicians are highly trained professionals who are handsomely compensated for their expertise. There would be no reason for them to engage in clandestine, illegal transplantations. On the contrary, they would have every incentive not to participate in such activities. If such illegal activities were detected—and they surely would be given the large number of people involved, the highly technical nature of the procedures, and the abhorrent nature of the alleged activities—this would mean the effective end of the surgeon or physician's career, with catastrophic financial and personal implications.

In sum, organ transplantation is such an immensely complicated, highly technical, heavily regulated, extremely time-sensitive procedure, involving so many highly trained professional personnel and so much sophisticated medical equipment, that clandestine organ trafficking is, quite simply, an impossibility from a practical point of view. The charges that children are being kidnapped and murdered for such purposes make the allegations even more dubious.

Nor is there any evidence that clandestine rings exist in order to kidnap children or others in order to extract their corneas for transplant. Corneas, which are tissues, not organs, can be extracted up to 12 hours after death for use in sight-restoring transplantations. This means that if anyone wished to procure corneas illicitly, they could do so by bribing someone at a morgue to extract corneas from corpses. There is no reason for anyone to kidnap or murder children or others in order to obtain corneas.

REPEATED INVESTIGATIONS FIND NO EVIDENCE FOR THE RUMOR

In early 1987, when the "baby parts" rumor first appeared, representatives of the U.S. Justice Department, the Federal Bureau of Investigation, the Food and Drug Administration, the National Institutes of Health, the Department of Health and Human Services, and the Immigration and Naturalization Service all investigated their records and stated that they had no evidence that would indicate alleged organ trafficking.

On July 23, 1987, in response to a European Parliament resolution asking for an investigation of such charges, the European Community Commission stated that it "does not know of any transplant operations performed in Europe for which the organs of Latin American children have been used."

On October 7, 1987, the Geneva-based non-governmental organization Defense for Children, International (DCI) stated, "In recent months, DCI has tried to have these reports verified by its representatives in Central America. So far, these investigations have failed to find any evidence to substantiate the reports."

On January 29, 1988, after these charges had resurfaced in Guatemala, the Director of the Treasury Police, Mr. Oscar Augusto Diaz Urquizu, stated: "The institution which I direct has no proof, evidence, or indication that Guatemalan children are being sent to the United States, or to any other country, to be dismembered and used as organ donors."

In a July 11, 1988 report, U.N. Secretary General Javier Perez de Cuellar warned that reports of such activities issued by the International Association of Democratic Lawyers were "possibly fictitious," adding that there has been no "corroboration" for them.

On August 23, 1988, Gene Pierce, Executive Director of the United Network for Organ Sharing, stated that, "since the establishment of the Scientific Registry on October 1, 1987, UNOS has kept very detailed records on organ donors. There has been no documentation of any Latin American children under the age of 5 becoming donors in the United States."

On August 25, 1988, Linda Sheaffer, Director of the Divison of Organ Transplantation at the U.S. Public Health Service, stated that such illegal transplants would be "not only impractical but impossible." She pointed out that some organ transplants "take up to 14 hours, none of the procedures could occur without the complete cooperation and knowledge of the hospital staff," and "any such large scale operation would not be kept secret."

On September 23, 1988, the Paris-based International Federation for Human Rights released a "Mission Report" on their "Investigation on Possible Trafficking in Infant Organs." It stated, "We have not been able to find a single piece of evidence indicating that such a trafficking operation is really occurring."

On September 26, 1988, the U.S. Federal Bureau of Investigation stated that "based on a review of all information available to the FBI, these charges are completely unfounded."

On October 3, 1988, R.C. Steiner, chief of the U.S. National Central Bureau, which represents the United States in the international criminal investigative organization Interpol, said that its records "do not reflect any requests for criminal investigative assistance from either the police in the United States or the police of any foreign country concerning this matter."

On October 8, 1988, Assistant Secretary of State Richard Schifter stated that "My government has made an exhaustive investigation of the charges and rumors related to this matter and both the U.S. Justice Department and the Federal Bureau of Investigation have concluded that they are totally groundless."

On November 18, 1988, Guatemala's Diario de Centro America reported that Guatemalan president Cerezo had stated: "The Guatemalan government has made serious and thorough investigations on the trafficking of babies and it has been concluded that the rumors on the 'butchering' of babies are false."

On June 6, 1989, Assistant Secretary for Health James Mason and Surgeon General C. Everett Koop released a lengthy letter in which they pointed out that "the technical and medical aspects of organ transplantation make it impossible to obtain and transplant organs secretly." They stated, "The requirements of the process, including numerous highly trained professional personnel and sophisticated equipment, assure that any such activity would be detected and exposed," stressing that "removals of organs is a complex surgical procedure, performed only in hospitals, and specialized technical arrangements are needed to preserve the organs." Mason and Koop went on to point out, "Organ transplant procedures are also highly complex and must be performed in the highest level surgical facilities, most often in large hospitals affiliated with schools for the education of physicians." "Because of the nature of the technology involved," they concluded, "these activities could not be conducted in secret or makeshift facilities."

On February 7, 1991, Eduardo Mestre Sarmiento, the Permanent Representative of Colombia to the United Nations in Geneva, sent a letter to Mr. Jan Martenson, U.N. Under-Secretary General, in which he stated that the office of the Attorney General of Colombia had launched an "exhaustive" investigation of charges made by the International Association of Democratic Lawyers that children's organs from Colombia were being sold. Mr. Mestre stated that the investigation had found that the claims made by IADL were "completely unsubstantiated," adding that "the newspapers referred to as having published the news item never had knowledge of these acts."

On July 20, 1992, the Mexican newspaper Epoca published the findings of its investigation of this issue. It stated:

Doctor Arturo Dib Kuri, director of the Health Secretariat's National Transplants Register, expresses this opinion: "The possibilities of human organ and tissue trafficking are extremely remote. It would be virtually impossible to conceal a criminal organization of this magnitude."

The interviewee continues: "First, to obtain an idea of what we are saying, I need only mention that, in the entire country, there would be, at the most, 10 doctors capable of performing a transplant. In an operation of this type, such as a liver transplant, 32 persons participate in an operating room, including doctors, nurses, paramedics, and team and technical personnel; not to mention laboratory workers and the personnel required for post-operative hospitalization. . . ."

Doctor Dib Kuri also describes the conditions for preserving an organ outside the body. The medical technique for extracting a kidney is very delicate.

"Organs such as the heart, lung, liver, and pancreas have, at the most, a duration of 6 hours after they are extracted from the human body; and this is under preservation conditions requiring advanced technology and an infrastructure that any hospital could hardly possess.'"It takes from 4 to 6 hours. . . . Once it is outside the donor's body, it must be kept at a temperature no lower than 4 degrees centigrade, because the organ must retain optimal oxygenation levels."

Dib Kuri comments:

"The number of persons engaged in a surgical practice of this type, and the complex hospital infrastructure that it requires, make it extremely difficult to keep this type of crime clandestine, in the event that anyone were to attempt to deal in organs."

"I can't imagine one of those 10 doctors that we have in Mexico who are capable of making a transplant becoming involved with a criminal organization engaged in such activities. These are not operations that can be performed in any old hospital."

"The recipient would not risk receiving an organ from anyone. All this is a mere rumor. I don't dare deny that there are stolen children, but it could be done for other purposes, such as prostitution; it is highly unlikely to be for the purpose of extracting and selling their organs."

On April 19, 1993, after Honduran Congresswoman Rosario Godoy de Osejo made accusations that "baby parts" trafficking was occurring in Honduras, the President of the Honduran Supreme Court, Orlando Lozano Martinez, stated: "These allegations have been coming forward for three years and we have not been able to prove anything nor find merit in them through investigation." On April 21, Honduran Attorney General Leonardo Matute Murillo stated that his office had investigated organ trafficking charges for more than one year and found nothing to support them. The spokesman for the Honduran police also stated that the police had investigated organ trafficking allegations and found them to be completely false.

On June 7, 1993, Mexico's El Financiero newspaper quoted Pablo Chapa, the director of complaints at Mexico City's attorney general's office, as stating, "I have not seen a single case where a person has been kidnapped and has later appeared with scars where his organs were taken, or his eyes were taken away. If these famous clandestine hospitals existed, we would have found out about them immediately." Dr. Arturo Dib Kuri, director of Mexico's National Registry of Transplants, stated, "I compare the rumor of stolen children whose organs are sold for transplant to a story saying that several thieves stole three [space] ships from Cape Canaveral to go to the moon."

In April 1996, French folklorist Veronique Campion-Vincent completed an extremely comprehensive 285-page study for the French Transplant Organization entitled Transplantation, Rumor, and the Media: Accounts of Organ Theft. Her voluminous and extremely thorough examination concluded unequivocally that organ theft rumors are an unfounded urban legend.

THE RUMOR'S ADVERSE IMPACTS

The false "baby parts" rumor has done tremendous damage in a number of different ways.

Most dramatically, it led to attacks on Americans and others in Guatemala during March 1994. On March 8, a mob in a Guatemalan town burned the police station in which an American wrongly suspected of child kidnapping had been held. The mob resisted the efforts of several hundred riot police and was not quieted until army troops and armored vehicles arrived to restore order. On March 29, an American tourist, June Weinstock, was savagely beaten by a mob, which accused her of abducting a Guatemalan child. A mob surrounded the building where Weinstock was being protected by local authorities, broke in, and dragged her out after a five-hour siege. Weinstock was pelted with rocks and beaten with pieces of firewood, suffering multiple broken bones, internal injuries, and severe head injuries that caused serious, long-term damage. She remains unable to speak or walk and requires 24-hour nursing care.

In addition to assaults on Americans, Guatemalan media reported numerous attempted lynchings by angry mobs that believed that "strangers" were allegedly stealing their children. A Swiss volcanologist, a Salvadoran family visiting relatives, foreign assistance workers, backpackers, and Guatemalan citizens all reportedly suffered such attacks.

The hysteria generated by this rumor has had an adverse impact on intercountry adoptions in a number of countries, according to adoption groups. In May 1991, the Turkish government announced that it was suspending intercountry adoptions because of the rumor. Adoptions have also been suspended or hindered in Honduras, Guatemala, Brazil, Mexico, and many other countries. As a result, some children who might have found loving homes remain in orphanages. The government of Bulgaria has even gone so far as to require prospective adoptive parents from foreign countries to sign a form stating, "I will not permit my child to be an organ donor nor allow the child to give organs or be a part of any medical experiments."

The rumor has also led to groundless, but widespread fears among parents in Latin America and elsewhere who believe that their child might be kidnapped for the purpose of organ transplantation.

Finally, the rumor is probably also causing an indirect but very real loss of life. Voluntary organ donation is a very altruistic activity, and one that can be adversely affected by any perception of impropriety or illicit behavior. Worldwide, there are long waiting lists for organ transplants that exceed donor supply and, as a result, people die every day because of the lack of sufficient donor organs. To the extent that the organ theft rumor has been believed, it has very likely decreased voluntary organ donation, and thereby caused many premature deaths.

1993: THE RUMOR IS GIVEN CREDENCE IN TELEVISION DOCUMENTARIES

In November 1993, two hour-long television documentaries, one British/Canadian and the other French, gave credence to the "baby parts" rumor. Both programs contained numerous errors.

The British/Canadian program, The Body Parts Business, featured the claim of an eight-year old Honduran child, Charlie Alvarado, that he had been kidnapped by people who said they intended to sell his organs. Alvarado claimed that he had escaped after four days of captivity.

What the program did not mention was that Alvarado identified a German and a Swiss volunteer who worked at local children's homes as his alleged kidnappers. Both were arrested and held for six days while the case was investigated. After the investigation, the judge dismissed the case as a fabrication. The boy could not remember the day on which he had allegedly been kidnapped and had no bruises from the ropes with which he claimed he had been tied.

The Body Parts Business also featured an interview with the family of Pedro Reggi, who had been a patient at the Montes de Oca mental institution in Argentina. In the film, it is alleged that Reggi was blinded when his corneas were forcibly removed.

A few days after the program was broadcast, Reggi and his half-brother appeared on the Argentine television program Hora Clave and retracted the allegation, stating that Reggi had lost his eyesight due to an "infection." A subsequent investigation revealed that he had suffered from "bilateral congenital cataracts" as an infant and had severe eye problems in the mid-1980s that were judged to be inoperable. He lost his eyesight due to disease.

The French program Organ Snatchers also highlighted the false Pedro Reggi claim. In addition, it wrongly suggested that clandestine organ trafficking might be occurring in the United States. The program's examination of the situation the United States, however, included no interviews with any transplant physicians or surgeons or anyone knowledgeable about the requirements of organ transplantation. The only person it included was a professor of women's studies and medical ethics who believed that clandestine organ trafficking might be occurring, but had no evidence of this.

The French program concluded with a dramatic sequence in which a mother in Colombia claimed that after she took her young son Jeison to a hospital for diarrhea, he emerged blind because his corneas had been stolen. The blind boy, misidentified as Jenson, was shown on the pages of Life magazine in October 1993, playing a flute.

On February 4, 1994, the Colombian government's Office of Human Rights issued a report on its investigation of these allegations. It stated that Jeison had gone blind due to disease. After he was admitted to a Colombian hospital in February 1983, at four months of age, he was found to be suffering from multiple illnesses, including "severe bilateral eye infection [which] had produced perforations of the corneas, conjunctivitis, and drainage of purulent matter from each of his corneas." The prognosis was for a total loss of vision, which, according to Jeison's medical records, occurred on February 23, 1983.

In short, the "revelations" of alleged organ and cornea trafficking in both programs turned out to be groundless.

PRESTIGIOUS INTERNATIONAL ORGANIZATIONS EXAMINE THE RUMOR

In addition to the media attention generated by the British/Canadian and French programs, both the European Parliament and United Nations have issued reports that have given credence to the "baby parts" rumor.

On February 25, 1993, the European Parliament issued a report on prohibiting trade in transplant organs that made many valuable suggestions but also included the unsubstantiated claim that "there is evidence that fetuses, children, and adults in some developing countries have been mutilated and others murdered with the aim of obtaining transplant organs for export to rich countries." The report, drafted by the former French Minister of Health and then-European Member of Parliament Leon Schwartzenberg, claimed that "to deny the existence of such trafficking is comparable to denying the existence of the ovens and gas chambers during the last war."

On September 14, 1993, The European Parliament adopted a resolution on prohibiting trade in transplant organs based on this report. In subsequent days, Mr. Schwartzenberg revealed that the source for most of his information had been an article in the August 1992 issue of *Le Monde Diplomatique*. This article was written by French journalist Maite Pinero, a former correspondent for the French communist newspaper L'Humanite, who, since April 1987, has written numerous articles that consistently give credence to organ theft allegations, even long after they have been repudiated or discredited. The claims in *Le Monde Diplomatique*, which Mr. Schwartzenberg repeated, were groundless.

A former U.N. Special Rapporteur on the Sale of Children, Vitit Muntarbhorn, also gave credence to the rumor in several reports he issued from 1991 to 1994. The Special Rapporteur depended largely on press accounts, which included many mistakes, and offered no credible evidence of trafficking in children's organs. In the June 26, 1995 issue of Newsweek, Myriam Tebourbi, a U.N. employee who assisted the Special Rapporteur, commented, "We never had any real evidence. He had lots of allegations, but nothing concrete. . . . We had no resources to mount our own investigation."

1994–1996: THE RUMOR ATTAINS UNPRECEDENTED CREDIBILITY

On March 7, 1994, Eric Sottas, director of the Geneva-based World Organization Against Torture, repeated various claims of "baby parts" trafficking in a 15-page paper that received wide publicity. Mr. Sottas also incorrectly stated that only one-fifth of U.S. organ transplants are centrally recorded and wrongly implied that organ sales are permitted in the United States. In fact, organ sales are illegal in the U.S. and all organ transplants are centrally recorded and monitored.

In May 1994, Spanish journalist Jose Manuel Martin Medem published a 200-page book Ninos de Repuesto (Spare-Parts Children), which credulously repeated many previous "baby parts" allegations. Despite researching the subject for six years, the author apparently did not realize that many of the charges he mentioned had been repudiated or disproved years earlier.

In January 1995, Eye Snatchers, an edited version of Organ Snatchers, was broadcast on M-6, a major television station in France. Eye Snatchers repeated the allegations about the Argentine youth Pedro Reggi and the Colombian child Jeison, both of which had been decisively disproved one year earlier. It made no mention of the fact that its main alleged "smoking gun" cases of cornea theft had been disproved. It simply ignored these facts as if they had not occurred.

In May 1995, Eye Snatchers received France's prestigious Albert-Londres prize in the audio-visual department, having been voted by a panel of journalists to be the best television program of the year in France.

The Colombian government was so outraged by the award of this prestigious journalism prize to a program that falsely accused Colombian doctors of stealing eyes from living children that it flew Jeison to Paris for an examination by a team of French doctors.

Jeison and his father arrived in Paris in August 1995 and the boy was examined by three prominent French doctors: Dr. Gilles Renard, of the Ophthalmological Service of the Hotel-Dieu Hospital; Dr. Marc Gentilini, of the Infectious and Tropical Diseases branch of the Pitie-Salpetriere Hospital; and Dr. Alain Fischer, of the Pediatric Immunology Service of Necker Hospital. The report on their examination of Jeison stated unequivocally that the boy had not had his eyes or corneas stolen. It reported that a stump of the eyeball and a number of fragments of corneal tissue remained in his eye sockets, proof that the corneas and the eye had not been removed. The condition of Jeison's eyes was exactly what would have been expected as a result of the disease from which he had suffered, as recorded in his medical records.

Shortly after this report was released, the panel that had awarded the Albert-Londres prize to Eye Snatchers decided to suspend the prize, pending further investigation.

Meanwhile, on March 18, 1996, a series of articles repeating "baby parts" claims in the Brazilian newspaper Correio Braziliense was awarded the "King of Spain" prize for journalism. The articles repeated the long-disproved Jeison and Pedro Reggi charges and many other false claims that had appeared in the world press. The series' author, Ana Beatriz Magno, admitted in the March 20 issue of the Spanish newspaper El Pais that "I can only reproduce what the international press has written" on this issue and that she did not seek to verify any of the claims she had repeated.

Also on March 20, 1996, the Albert-Londres panel in France decided to reaffirm its award to Eye Snatchers, although with numerous "reservations." The panel criticized the program for having been "too categorical" in its allegations of cornea theft, which it admitted that the great majority of ophthalmologists thought were groundless, and admonished the program's producer, Marie-Monique Robin, for having "allowed herself to be carried away with emotion," for having made "unnecessarily injurious judgments," and for having been insufficiently skeptical of the claims of cornea theft. Despite these many criticisms, the panel nevertheless reaffirmed its award of the prize. In its statement, the panel did not address, or indicate that it had sought to examine, most of the errors in the program. Instead, it appears to have focused almost exclusively on Jeison case, which had been hotly contested in France. Commenting on the panel's decision, the French magazine Telerama wondered: "How is it possible for the Albert Londres jury to justify the award of its prize to an investigation that they themselves judge to have little reliability?"

CONCLUSION

Despite the fact that it is totally unfounded, the "baby parts" rumor is now perceived as fact and accepted as conventional wisdom in large parts of the world. It has generated hysteria in Central American countries, led to brutal, unprovoked attacks on Americans and others, disrupted the lives of numerous prospective adoptive parents and the children they wished to adopt, won prestigious media awards in Europe, caused major disruptions in cornea donations in Latin America, and is, in all likelihood, causing numerous premature deaths because of its adverse effects on organ donation.

This sensationalistic rumor springs from deep, irrational, but very powerful anxieties stirred by advances in the life-saving process of organ transplantation. These fears have unfortunately been fanned by some who have cynically advanced this rumor for political purposes. The false rumor has also been propagated by many others who genuinely believe it. As a result of this cycle of events, the "baby parts" myth has now attained such widespread currency that it continues to feed on itself and, tragically, is widely believed despite numerous corrective statements, authoritative statements pointing to the impossibility of such practices occurring, and the fact that despite almost ten years of searching, no government, non-governmental organization, intergovernmental body, or investigative journalist has ever produced any credible evidence to support the charges.

DONATION & TRANSPLANTATION MYTHS [AS LISTED BY OPTN AT HTTP://WWW.OPTN.ORG/ABOUT/ MYTHS.ASP]

There is a severe organ shortage in this country. Despite continuing efforts at public education, misconceptions and inaccuracies about donation persist. It's a tragedy if even one person decides against donation because they don't know the truth. Following is a list of the most common myths along with the actual facts:

Myth: If emergency room doctors know you're an organ donor, they won't work as hard to save you.

Fact: If you are sick or injured and admitted to the hospital, the number one priority is to save your life. Organ donation can only be considered after brain death has been declared by a physician. Many states have adopted legislation allowing individuals to legally designate their wish to be a donor should brain death occur, although in many states Organ Procurement Organizations also require consent from the donor's family. See the Donor Designation Fact Sheet to learn more about legislation in your area.

Myth: When you're waiting for a transplant, your financial or celebrity status is as important as your medical status.

Fact: When you are on the transplant waiting list for a donor organ, what really counts is the severity of your illness, time spent waiting, blood type, and other important medical information.

Myth: Having "organ donor" noted on your driver's license or carrying a donor card is all you have to do to become a donor.

Fact: While a signed donor card and a driver's license with an "organ donor" designation are legal documents, organ and tissue donation is usually discussed with family members prior to the donation. To ensure that your family understands your wishes, it is important that you tell your family about your decision to donate LIFE.

Myth: Only hearts, livers, and kidneys can be transplanted.

Fact: Needed organs include the heart, kidneys, pancreas, lungs, liver, and intestines. Tissue that can be donated include the eyes, skin, bone, heart valves and tendons.

Myth: Your history of medical illness means your organs or tissues are unfit for donation.

Fact: At the time of death, the appropriate medical professionals will review your medical and social histories to determine whether or not you can be a donor. With recent advances in transplantation, many more people than ever before can be donors. It's best to tell your family your wishes and sign up to be an organ and tissue donor on your driver's license or an official donor document. See the Donor Designation Fact Sheet to learn more about legislation in your state.

Myth: You are too old to be a donor.

Fact: People of all ages and medical histories should consider themselves potential donors. Your medical condition at the time of death will determine what organs and tissue can be donated.

Myth: If you agree to donate your organs, your family will be charged for the costs.

Fact: There is no cost to the donor's family or estate for organ and tissue donation. Funeral costs remain the responsibility of the family.

Myth: Organ donation disfigures the body and changes the way it looks in a casket.

Fact: Donated organs are removed surgically, in a routine operation similar to gallbladder or appendix removal. Donation does not change the appearance of the body for the funeral service.

Myth: Your religion prohibits organ donation.

Fact: All major organized religions approve of organ and tissue donation and consider it an act of charity.

Myth: There is real danger of being heavily drugged, then waking to find you have had one kidney (or both) removed for a black market transplant.

Fact: This tale has been widely circulated over the Internet. There is absolutely no evidence of such activity ever occurring in the U.S. While the tale may sound credible, it has no basis in the reality of organ transplantation. Many people who hear the myth probably dismiss it, but it is possible that some believe it and decide against organ donation out of needless fear.

Timeline for
Transplantation Issues

500 BC   Apocryphal account relates that Chinese physician Pien Chi'ia transplanted the hearts between two warriors to give each the strengths that the other did not possess.

c. 400 BC   The first grafting of skin flaps for facial reconstruction of noses and ears may date as far back as 800 BC but is generally thought to have occurred around 400 BC, as indicated in reports by the Indian surgeon Susrata, or Sushruta, in his medical treatise *Susrata Samhita*, or *Sushruta Samita*.

100–300   Once again, apocryphal accounts of transplantation arise, including the reattachment of a soldier's hand by Saint Mark in the first century and then the replacement of an amputated leg of a Roman with the leg of an Ethiopian gladiator by the Christian physicians, martyrs, and brothers Saint Cosmos and Saint Damien some time in the second century.

200   Noted Chinese surgeon Hua-To of the Han Dynasty makes the first reference to the concept of organ transplantation as a possible medical therapy for replacing diseased organs with healthy ones.

1600   The father of modern plastic surgery, Gaspare Tagliacozzi, or Tagliocozzi, transplants the skin from patients' arms to repair their damaged noses and ears.

1688   The first successful bone graft is reported, involving the use of bone from a dog's skull to help repair a damaged human cranium.

1740s   French physician Garengeot reports grafting a soldier's nose back on using skin from another part of the soldier's body.

1744   Swiss medical researcher Abraham Tremply performs first animal transplant experiments using hydras, small organisms that are often less than an inch (2.5 cm) long; Charles Bonnet, a French philosopher and scientists, confirms successful transplant experiments in animals with his research using earthworms.

1749   French naturalist and physiologist Henri-Louis Duhamel du Monceau successfully transplants spurs removed from young chickens onto the comb of the same animal and onto other chickens.

1804   Giuseppe Boronio successfully grafts skin from one sheep onto the back of another sheep.

1869   Swiss surgeon Jacques Louis Reverdin performs first successful fresh skin allograft, that is, the transplantation of one person's tissue to another person, noting that successful grafts required use of thinner tissues

1900–1914   Numerous transplant experiments in dogs take place, including autografts (from the same dog), allografts (between different dogs), and xenografts (between dogs and other animals).

1906   Physician Edward Zim performs the first corneal transplant.

1906   French physician Mathieu Jaboulay makes an early but unsuccessful attempt at a kidney (renal) transplantation between humans.

1909   First human xenotransplant (transplantation between different species) occurs when Ernst Unger transplants an ape's kidney to a young girl, whose death convinces Unger that a nonsurgical, biological barrier exists to prevent successful transplantations.

1920s   Controversy arises as a charlatan in Kansas named John Romulus Brinkley falsely claims that inserting glands from a virile goat into the testicles of men will give the men sexual potency.

1954   First successful human kidney transplant takes place when Dr. Joseph E. Murray and colleagues at the Peter Bent Brigham Hospital (now Brigham & Women's Hospital) in Boston transplants a kidney from Ronald Herrick into his identical twin Richard, who went on to live for eight more years.

1958   French physician Jean Dausset describes first leukocyte antigen, which leads to tissue matching beyond blood types.

1962   Surgeons at Peter Bent Brigham Hospital perform the first cadaveric liver transplant.

1963   Thomas Starzl performs the first liver transplant at the University of Colorado, and James Hardy performs the first lung transplant at the University of Mississippi.

1967   Christian Bernaard performs the first heart transplant at Groote Schur Hospital in Cape Town, South Africa. His removal of a heart from a "brain dead" donor leads to ethical concerns over transplantation and how organs should be harvested. Thomas Starzl performs first successful liver transplant.

1969–1974 Thomas Starzl conducts the first transplants of nonhuman primate livers into children, with survival rates ranging from one day to two weeks.

1979   David Sutherland performs the first living-related pancreas transplant in Minnesota.

1983   The U.S. Food and Drug Administration approves use of the drug cyclosporine, making it the first drug to treat organ rejection by suppressing the human immune system.

1983   The debate over buying and selling organs garners national attention when a Virginia company announces plans to buy and sell human organs, with a price of up to $10,000 to be paid for a kidney. The plan never comes to fruition because the medical community and legislators quickly express outrage and proceed to initiate laws and guidelines to prohibit the marketing of organs.

1984   Baby Fae is the first infant to receive a xenotransplant when a walnut-sized baboon heart is transplanted into the infant, who lived for twenty-one days.

1985   The Ethics Committee of the Council of the Transplantation Society issues guidelines prohibiting the practice of buying and selling organs.

1986   The United Network for Organ Sharing (UNOS) obtains the federal contract to make certain that organs are allocated fairly and to set membership criteria and standards for transplant centers.

1988   The Joint Commission on Accreditation of Health Care Organizations (JCAHO) sets donor identification and notification standards that require hospitals to have identification, referral, and organ and tissue procurement procedures put in place.

1990   Vaughn A. Starnes performs the first successful living-related lung transplant at the Stanford University Medical Center.

1991   The first successful small intestine transplant is performed.

1993   A national survey by Gallup indicates that more than 80 percent of people in the United States support organ and tissue donation.

1994   National Coalition on Donation collaborates with the Advertising Council to develop an ongoing national public education campaign designed to increase organ and tissue donations, which are severely lagging behind patient needs.

1995   Questions arise and the public expresses concern over the fairness of organ allocation when baseball legend Mickey Mantle quickly receives a donor organ to replace his failing liver.

1996   Congress passes the organ Donation Insert Card Act, authorizing income tax refund mailings to include information about organ and tissue donation.

1998   Amadeo Marcus performs the first successful living-donor liver transplant at the medical College of Virginia.

1998   James Thomson of the University of Wisconsin at Madison becomes the first scientist to isolate and culture human embryonic stem cells, which has led to moral, ethical, and political controversies concerning the use of such cells for transplantation therapies.

1999   The U.S. Department of Health and Human Services issues the amended "Final Rule" for organ and procurement and transplantation, including stipulations calling for broader and more equitable sharing of organs.

2001   President George W. Bush makes speech limiting federal funding of research with embryonic stem cells to those "cell lines" already in existence.

2002   PPL Therapeutics, Inc., creates the world's first cloned pigs lacking the gene for the galactose sugar, which is associated with hyperacute, or immediate, rejection. This advance increases the possibility of one day performing a successful xenotransplantation between pigs and humans.

2002   Michael Hurewitz dies only three days after donating a portion of his liver to his brother Adam, who went on to recover fully. Hurewitz's death brings to the forefront the ethical issues concerning whether it is right for the medical community to jeopardize a healthy person's life in order to save another.

2005   The U.S. Food and Drug Administration approves the first ever transplant of fetal stem cells into human brains. The cells are to be transplanted into children suffering from the deadly Batten disease.

2005   French surgeons perform the first partial face transplant onto a woman who had been disfigured by a dog bite. Concerns over protocol and the ethics of such a surgery quickly ensue.

2006   On July 18, 2006, the U.S. Congress passed legislation with a vote of 63-37 that would have lifted restrictions on government funding for embryonic stem cell research imposed by President Bush in 2001. The following day, Bush vetoed the bill, exercising his veto powers for the first time in his more than five years in office.

Glossary

Acute rejection Rejection of a transplanted organ or tissue that usually occurs in the first year and is due to an immunological attack on the grafted tissues.

Allocation The process of determining how organs are to be distributed according to specific policies and guidelines designed to ensure an equitable, ethical, and medically appropriate approach to the process.

Allograft A graft or transplant between two individuals of the same species but of different genetic makeup; sometimes referred to as allotransplantation.

Antibody A protein produced by the body's immune system to fight off foreign invaders such as bacteria and, in the case of transplantation, allograft organs.

Antigen A foreign molecule or substance usually found on the surface of a cell, such as cells that make up a transplant, that can initiate an immune response.

Autograft A graft of skin or other tissue that is taken from the body of the person and then grafted onto another part of the same person's body.

Brain death A state in which a person is deemed to have irreversible stoppage of cerebral and brain stem function.

Cadaveric donor organ An organ obtained from an individual who has recently died of causes that do not affect the resumed functioning of the transplanted organ.

Chronic rejection A slow process of organ or tissue rejection in which the host immune system conducts a continuous immunological attack on the transplanted organ, likely resulting in the eventual loss of organ function.

Crossmatch test A test in which donor and recipient blood samples are mixed together to determine whether the donor and recipient are compatible for an allograft transplant. A positive crossmatch means that the potential recipient has antibodies against the donor's antigens, making them incompatible. A negative crossmatch means that there is no reaction and the transplant can proceed.

Cyclosporine An immunosuppressive drug.

Diastolic The bottom of two blood pressure numbers, which measures blood pressure when the heart is at rest.

Donor An individual who provides an organ for transplantation into someone else.

Donor registries Confidential databases of registered organ donors.

Glucose A type of sugar found in the blood.

Graft An organ or tissue that is transplanted.

Graft rejection An attempt by the immune system to reject or destroy the "foreign" organ or tissue.

Histocompatibility A term that refers to the similarity of tissue between different individuals. The condition in which the cells of one tissue can survive in the presence of cells of another tissue. In the case of transplantation, histocompatibility is determined through the examination of human leukocyte antigens (HLA) and is often referred to as "tissue typing." The process helps to decrease the likelihood of a patient "rejecting" a transplanted organ.

Human leukocyte antigens (HLA) A genetically determined series of antigens that are present on human white blood cells and tissues.

Immune system The biological system that protects the body from invasion by foreign substances, such as bacteria and viruses, and from cancer cells.

Immunosuppression The reduction of immune system functioning to prevent a reaction against donor marrow or stem cells and to prevent GVHD.

Immunosuppressive drugs (immunosuppressants) Antirejection medications provided to suppress the immune system and prevent rejection of a transplanted organ.

Informed consent A process in which patients are given enough information to understand and consent to a medical or surgical treatment or to participate in a clinical trial or other medical research with a full understanding of the risks involved.

Islet cell transplant The transplantation of cells called Islets of Langerhans, which are found in the pancreas and which secrete hormones such as insulin and glucagon into the blood.

Living related donor (LRD) A blood relative who donates an organ to a recipient.

Living unrelated donor A tissue or organ donor who is not a blood relative of the recipient.

Match A general term denoting the compatibility between a recipient and a donor based primarily on HLA typing.

Pathology Deviation from a healthy or normal condition; the medical specialty that studies the causes, nature, and effects of disease.

Organ preservation The process of preserving organs from the time that they are taken from the donor's body until they are transplanted into the patient.

Organ Procurement Organization (OPO) Organizations responsible for the retrieval, preservation, and transportation of organs for transplantation.

Rejection An immune response against grafted tissue, which, if not successfully treated, results in failure of the graft to survive.

Renal Refers to the kidney.

Stem cells An embryonic or primitive cell that can lead to the development of all types of specialized cells.

Tissue A group or organization of similar cells, such as blood, bones, or bone marrow, that perform a special function.

Tissue typing A blood test completed before transplantation to evaluate the closeness of tissue match between donor's organ and recipient's HLA antigens.

Xenograft An organ or tissue transplanted from one species into another.

Xenotourism A term referring to the potential for patients to travel to foreign countries for the express purpose of obtaining a xenograft or associated therapy that is not available in their own countries.

Xenotransplantation Transplantation of organs and tissues between individuals of different species.

Xenozoonosis The transmission of infectious disease from animal to human, particularly through the transplantation of an animal tissue or organ into a human.

Further Reading

Abul-Fotouh, Muhammad Yehia Ahmad. 1987. "Sale of Human Organs in the Balance of Legitimacy." Medical Jurisprudence Third Symposium: "The Islamic Vision of Some Medical Practices," Islamic Organization for Medical Sciences. Islam Set Web site, http://www.islamset.com/bioethics/vision/my_abulfotouh.html

Ad Hoc Committee of the Harvard Medical School to Examine the Definition of Brain-death. 1968. "Guidelines for the determination of death. Report of the Ad Hoc Committee of the Harvard Medical School to Examine the Definition of Brain-death." *Journal of the American Medical Association*, 205, 337–340.

Altman, Lawrence K. 2004, December 21. "The Ultimate Gift: 50 Years of Organ Transplants," *New York Times*, p. F1.

Barclay, Laurie. 2004. "Brokering Organ Transplant on the Internet Raises Ethical Issues." Medscape Web site, http://www.medscape.com

BBC News Online. 2001. "Surgeons Sever Transplant Hand." BBC News Online Web site, http://news.bbc.co.uk/1/hi/world/europe/1151553.stm

Burdick, James F., et al. 1993. *Preferred Status For Organ Donors: A Report of the United Network for Organ Sharing Ethics Committee*. United Network for Organ Sharing Web site, http://www.unos.org/Resources/bioethics.asp?index=3

Bush, George. 2001. "The President Discusses Stem Cell Research." White House press release. The White House Web site, http://www.whitehouse.gov/news/releases/2001/08/20010809-2.html

Calandrillo, Steve P. 2004. "Cash for Kidneys? Utilizing Incentives to End America's Organ Shortage." *George Mason Law Review*, 13, 69.

Childress, James F. 1996. *Bulletin of the American College of Surgeons*, 81(3). American College of Surgeons Web site, http://www.facs.org/education/ethics/childresslect.html

Coalition for the Advancement of Medical Research. 2001. *"Survey Finds Overwhelming Public Support for Federal Funding of Stem Cell Research: Backing Comes from a Spectrum of Religious Affiliations and Ethical Perspectives,"* The Coalition for the Advancement of Medical Research press release. American Society of Reproductive Medicine Web site, http://lobby.la.psu.edu/_107th/121_Human_Cloning/Organizational_Statements/ASRM/ASRM_cloning_update_05_24_01.htm.

Concar, David. 2004, May 29. "The Boldest Cut." *New Scientist*, 32.

Doyle, Alden M., et al. 2004. "Organ Transplantation: Halfway through the First Century." *Journal of the American Society of Nephrology*, 15, 2965–2971.

Fox, Claude Earl. 1998, April 8. "House Testimony: National Organ Transplantation Policy." Health and Human Services Administration press release. Health and Human Services Web site, http://newsroom.hrsa.gov/speeches/foxOPTN.htm

Fox, Renee C., and Judith P. Swazey. 1992. *Spare Parts: Organ Replacement in American Society.* New York: Oxford University Press.

Galandiuk, Susan, and Sylvester Sterioff. 2005. "The Problems of Organ Donor Shortage." *Mayo Clinic Proceedings*, 880, 320–321.

Gottlieb, Agnes Hooper, et al. 1998. *1,000 years, 1,000 People: Ranking the Men and Women Who Shaped the Millennium.* New York: Kodansha International.

"Guidelines for the determination of death. Report of the medical consultants on the diagnosis of death to the President's Commission for the Study of Ethical Problems in Medicine and Biomedical and Behavioral Research." 1981. *Journal of the American Medical Association*, 246, 2184–2186.

Hastings Center. 1985. Ethical, Legal and Policy Issues Pertaining to Solid Organ Procurment. A Report of the Project on Organ Transplantation. Hastings Center Report.

Kahn, Jeffrey P., and Francis L. Delmonico. 2004. "The Consequences of Public Policy to Buy and Sell Organs for Transplantation." *American Journal of Transplantation*, 4(2), 178–180.

Kaserman, David L., and A. H. Barnett. 2002. The U.S. Organ Procurement System: A Prescription for Reform, Washington, DC: AEI Press.

King, L. P, et al. 2005. "Health Insurance and Cardiac Transplantation: A Call for Reform." *Journal of the American College of Cardiology*, 45, 1388–1391.

Kishore, R. R. 2005. "Human Organs, Scarcities, and Sale: Morality Revisited." *Journal of Medical Ethics*, 31, 362–365.

Kuhse, Helga, and Peter Singer. 1998. *A Companion to Bioethics.* Malden, MA: Blackwell Publishers, p. 332.

Langer, Gary. 2001, "Public Backs Stem Cell Research: Most Say Government Should Fund Use of Embryos." ABC News Web site, http://www.abcnews.go.com/sections/politics/DailyNews/poll010626.htm.

Matas, A. J., and M. Schnitzler. 2004. "Payment for Living Donor (Vendor) Kidneys: A Cost-Effectiveness Analysis." *American Journal of Transplantation*, 4(2), 216–221.

Mayes, Gwen. 2005. "A Rational Approach to Organ Allocation in 2005." Medscape Web site, http://www.medscape.com/viewarticle/507127

Mistichelli, Judith Adams. 1985. "Baby Fae: Ethical Issues Surrounding Cross-Species Transplantation." The Joseph and Rose Kennedy Institute of Ethics. *Scope Note*, 5, 19.

National Kidney Foundation. 2004. "Celebrating 50 Years of Transplantation." Kidney Foundation Web site, http://www.kidney.org

Neylan, John. 1997. "Enhancing Transplantation Medicine in the United States." American Society of Transplantation Web site, http://www.a-s-t.org/Public Policy/Library_htmls/neylants.htm

Office of the Inspector General. 1991. *The Distribution of Organs for Transplantation. Expectations and Practices (HHS) Publication No. OE-1-01-89-0050.* Washington, DC: Office of Analysis and Inspections.

O'Rourke, Devin D., and Philip Boyle, eds. 1993. *Medical Ethics: Sources of Catholic Teaching.* Washington, DC: Georgetown University Press.

Parmly, Michael E. 2001. "Sale of Human Organs in China." Hearing Before the Subcommittee on International Operations and Human Rights, House International Relations, Washington, DC. Department of State Web site, http://www.state.gov/g/drl/rls/rm/2001/3792.htm

Petechuk, David. 2005, Spring. "Transplantation Celebrates 50th." MATCH 3 [Thomas E. Starzl Transplantation Institute newsletter].

Pew Research Center for the People and the Press. 2005. "More See Benefits of Stem Cell Research: Opinions Divide Along Religious Lines." Pew Research Center for the People and the Press press release. Pew Research Center for the People and the Press Web site, http://people-press.org/commentary/display.php3?AnalysisID=111.

Public Broadcasting Service. 2003. "Xenotransplantation." *Religion and Ethics Newsweekly*, episode no. 621. Public Broadcasting Service Web site, http://www.pbs.org/wnet/religionandethics/week621/cover.html

Reams, Bernard D., Jr. 1984. *The National Organ Transplant Act of 1984: A Legislative History of Pub. L. No. 100-93* [i.e. Pub. L. No. 98-507]. Buffalo, NY: W.S. Hein.

Research America. 2005. "American Speak Out on Stem Cell Research." Research America Web site, http://www.researchamerica.org/polldata/.

Smith, Craig S. 2005, December 3. "Dire Wounds, a New Face, a Glimpse in a Mirror." *New York Times*, p. A1, A8.

Starzl, Thomas E. 1992. *The Puzzle People: Memoirs of a Transplant Surgeon.* Pittsburgh, PA: University of Pittsburgh Press.

Tabarrok, Alexander. 2004. "Life-Saving Incentives: Consequences, Costs and Solutions to Organ Shortage." Library of Economics and Liberty Web site, http://www.econlib.org/library/Columns/y2004/Tabarrokorgans.html

Tagliacozzi, Gaspare. 1597. *De Curtorum Chirurgia per Insitionem.*

Task Force on Organ Transplantation. 1986. *Organ Transplantation: Issues and Recommendations.* Washington, DC: U.S. Department of Health and Human Services.

Thompson, W. G. 1890. "Successful Brain Grafting." *New York Medical Journal*, 51, 701–702.

Tilney, Nicholas L. 2003. *Transplant: From Myth to Reality.* New Haven, CT: Yale University Press.

Truog, Robert D. 2005. "The Ethics of Organ Donation by Living Donors." *New England Journal of Medicine*, 353, 444–446.

UNOS Sharing Ethics Committee Payment Subcommittee. 1993. "Financial Incentives for Organ Donation." United Network for Organ Sharing Web site, http://www.optn.org/resources/bioethics.asp?index=3

Weiss, R. 2003, May 8. "400,000 Human Embryos Frozen in U.S." *Washington Post*, p. A10.

World Health Organization. 1991. "Guiding Principles on Human Organ Transplantation." World Health Organization Web site, http://www.who.int/ethics/topics/transplantation_guiding_principles/en/index1.html

Organizations and Web Resources

American Society of Minority Health and Transplant Professionals http://www.asmhtp.org/ This is a multicultural organization that serves health and transplant professionals by providing leadership in a national capacity on matters of diversity facing the transplant industry.

American Society of Transplant Surgeons (ASTS) http://www.asts.org This international society of surgeons takes a wide approach to fostering transplantation, including guiding those who make the policy decisions that influence the practice and science of transplantation and increasing organ donation.

Association of Organ Procurement Organizations (AOPO) http://www.aopo.org This organization includes federally certified OPOs who are members of the Organ Procurement and Transplantation Network and international members located from outside of the United States who are engaged in the promotion of organ and tissue donation.

Coalition on Donation http://www.shareyourlife.org This organization provides general information about organ and tissue donation, including how to become an organ and tissue donor.

Living Organ Donor.org http://www.livingorgandonor.org This organization is dedicated to providing the most current information for people considering being a living donor of a solid organ—such as a kidney or a lobe of a liver or lung. It is also for those who may be considering receiving an organ or who are waiting for a living organ transplant.

National Donor Family Council (NDFC) http://www.kidney.org/recips/donor The council provides information and resources for families of donors. It has more than 10,000 donor family and professional members.

National Minority Organ Tissue Transplant Education Program (MOTTEP) http://www.nationalmottep.org The program provides comprehensive information about minority health issues relating to donation and transplantation.

National Transplant Assistance Fund http://www.transplantfund.org This organization helps people raise money in their communities to cover uninsured medical expenses related to transplantation and catastrophic injury.

Organ Procurement and Transplantation Network (OPTN) http://www.optn.org The OPTN is the unified transplant network established by the United States Congress under the National Organ Transplant Act (NOTA) of 1984. It links all of the professionals involved in the donation and transplantation system.

The Partnership for Organ Donation http://www.transweb.org/partnership This independent, nonprofit organization is dedicated to saving and improving lives by closing the gap between the number of organ transplants that are possible and the number of organ transplants that actually occur.

Scientific Registry of Transplant Recipients (SRTR) http://www.ustransplant.org The SRTR supports the ongoing evaluation of the scientific and clinical status of solid organ transplantation in the United States. It is administered by the University Renal Research and Education Association (URREA) with the University of Michigan and provides extensive data on donation and transplantation.

South-Eastern Organ Procurement Foundation (SEOPF) http://www.seopf.org The oldest organ procurement organization in the United States was founded in 1969. Its mission is to enhance the donation, procurement, and transplantation of organs and tissues through scientific studies and professional education. SEOPF has been dedicated to serving the medical community as an educational resource. In 2006 SEOPF became the American Foundation for Donation & Transplantation.

Transplant Recipient International Organization (TRIO) http://www.trioweb.org This independent, nonprofit, international organization is committed to improving the quality of life of transplant candidates, recipients, their families, and the families of organ and tissue donors. TRIO serves its members in the following areas: Awareness, Support, Education, and Advocacy.

Transplant Week http://www.transplantweek.org This Web site provides the latest news about transplantation.

United Network for Organ Sharing (UNOS) http://www.unos.org This nonprofit, scientific, and educational organization administers the only Organ Procurement and Transplantation Network (OPTN) in the United States, which was established by the U.S. Congress in 1984.

Websites Associated with Organ and Tissue Donation and Transplantation http://www.argonet.co.uk/body/lnks.html Provides a comprehensive list of known sources of support and information about organ donation and transplantation. It targets almost every level of interest in the field, from professional to the general public, and has an international focus.

INDEX

ABOUT THE AUTHOR

DAVID PETECHUK is the author of *The Respiratory System* in Green-wood Press's Human Body Systems series, and the editor of the quarterly newsletter of the Thomas A. Starzl Transplantation Institute.

.